NAKED IN 30 DAYS:

A One-Month Guide to Getting Your Body, Mind and Spirit in Shape

THERESA ROEMER

For more information contact:
Riverdale Avenue Books
5676 Riverdale Avenue
Riverdale, NY 10471.
www.riverdaleavebooks.com

Design by www.formatting4U.com
Cover Design by Scott Carpenter
Photography by Jordan Matter

Digital ISBN 978-1-62601-252-3
Print ISBN 978-1-62601-253-0

All information presented within this book is intended for entertainment and educational purposes. Any health, diet or exercise advice is not intended as a medical diagnosis or treatment. The information in this book is not intended for people under 18 years of age, pregnant or breast feeding women, underweight individuals or people with eating disorders or any health condition that requires a special diet or mobility restrictions. We do not guarantee that the information will be completely accurate. Therefore the author, publisher and/or owners cannot be held responsible for any errors, omissions or inaccuracies published. The author and publisher recommend that you consult with a qualified doctor prior to starting any diet or exercise routine.

First Edition March 2016

Dedication

This book is dedicated to my son, Michael; my brother, Brian; and my father, Louis, who have always inspired me to be my best;

To my loving husband, Lamar, who has been the most supportive and encouraging partner throughout our marriage;

To my daughter, Tashina, and my twin grandsons, Zach and Zane, who keep me on my toes in the best possible way;

And to all the men and women who know deep in their hearts that they can defy the odds and change their lives.

Paula Conway, J.P. Hoornstra, Stacy Callahan and John Conway contributed to the writing and reporting in this book.

Table of Contents

Foreword

by Dr. George Davis

As Theresa Roemer's physician, I am sure you expect me to write this foreword as an affirmation of her fitness and diet plan and tell you that if you follow the instructions in these pages, you'll become fit and trim in 30 days.

But this book is more than that.

If you follow the insights and directions in this book, and make a commitment to lead a life of wellness, this book can change, and maybe even save, your life.

You see, before my physician wife and I opened our wellness center in Houston, I was trained as an emergency room doctor. Throughout my career, I have worked in many different ERs, and I see the same story again and again. The people I treat day in and day out do not come to me to find out how to live better and longer. They are already struggling to get to their next day when I see them. The patients that come into the emergency room are the product of years of bad nutrition and often bad life choices, and I found myself asking, is there any way to prevent this? That's why we started our wellness center.

But there was a personal reason too.

As much as my wife and I vowed to live a healthy life as the parents of two children, we let them off the hook more often than not. It is really hard to ask a child to give up gluten and sugar, so we were lenient.

Until two and a half years ago, when our 12-year-old daughter began suffering from autoimmune thyroiditis, a horrific disease that affects growth in puberty. We watched as our daughter had increasing lethargy, worsening grades and increasing weight, and we knew that if we continued to watch her decline, she would not have a very happy childhood and have many health issues to come. We decided to put her on the gluten-free diet we were on. Her condition was reversed and she continues on a gluten-free diet to this day. She is growing up to be a beautiful young lady and is enjoying her teenage years! Over time, we all learned that when we eat wrong, there's a price to pay.

Since then, the whole family has gone on the diet, and we are all happier and healthier!

So this book is my wellness plan that I have shared with Theresa, but also with my own wife and kids.

And, I'm not just a doctor, I'm on it too.

George Davis, MD FACEP
Board Certified Emergency Medicine

NAKED IN 30 DAYS: PART ONE

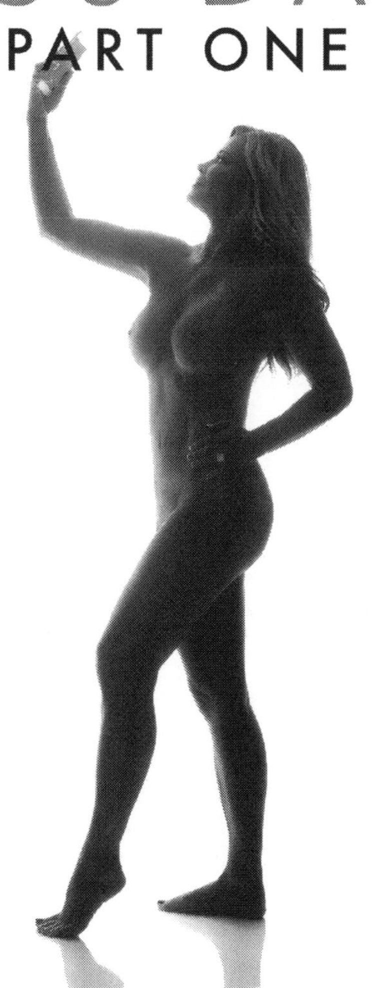

Introduction

It hasn't stopped hurting.

There I was, crying side-by-side with my mother at the funeral for my son, Michael. He was only 19 years old, the victim of a fatal car crash.

In some ways, he was my favorite child. He always had the power to make me smile when it seemed impossible. I can still remember the day I backed my car out of the driveway, the day my divorce became official in Michael's heart if not on paper. I looked in my rearview mirror and there he was, all of five years old, running down the street after my car. Of course I stopped, got out, and gave him a hug. Michael handed me a photo of him eating a watermelon. "Mommy," he said, "I never want you to forget what I look like."

My mother knew exactly how I felt the day Michael died.

Growing up on a ranch with my three siblings, my younger brother Brian was my closest ally. Unlike my two sisters, I was a tomboy. I joined Brian playing with our trucks, climbing trees, sliding down into the haystacks and playing in the cow tanks. He fed my inner tomboy, and I repaid the favor when we were older by getting him into weightlifting. We were best friends. We even had our children six weeks apart so each child would have a cousin their same age. When the air force showed up on my doorstep to tell me Brian had died of a massive heart attack overseas in England, I was in disbelief. "You're lying—his body is a temple," I thought. What I didn't know—what the air force didn't even know—was that Brian had lived his entire life with an undetected heart condition. That was the first time I experienced the pain of a loved one dying. As a big sister, I felt as if I had let my brother down. I hadn't protected him. Never again would I see the person who helped me be who I am. Brian was only 23.

I could only imagine how our mother felt that day, until I lost Michael. Then I knew. My mother turned to me and said, "I never wanted you to experience this pain."

***

I've been through hell and back. If it weren't for fitness and my faith in God, I wouldn't be here today. The easier response to each tragedy would've been to fall into a hole of depression, turn to drugs or alcohol, and stop taking care of myself when the pain became too much to bear. But somewhere along the way it dawned on me that fitness and taking care of your body can change your life. Diet and exercise won't solve all your personal problems, but being healthy makes you feel better. Then, with proper upkeep, you can defy long odds. I'm living proof.

The inspiration for this book really started before I was born. It seemed I had some illness every year from the time I arrived premature, which presented more problems a generation ago than it does now. I had rheumatic fever four times between ages four and 16 as a result of strep throat gone untreated. Our ranch was miles from town and we didn't run to the doctor when something was wrong. My parents would give me a homemade childhood remedy of honey, bourbon and lemon paired with Vicks VapoRub, then run a vaporizer. It didn't work.

When I would get sick enough, we would go to the children's hospital in Omaha, Nebraska, where I was told my heart had been weakened by my illnesses and I would never be a "normal child." The doctors told me I would never have any energy, my heart was too weak for sports, and I definitely wouldn't be able to have children.

To a small child, this felt like a death sentence. The thought of these doctors telling me I wouldn't be anything, and I couldn't do anything, made me start playing every sport imaginable. Turns out, I was good. I lettered in every sport you could think of—and no one in my family had ever been athletic. By the time I was 18, I was taken off my daily doses of penicillin. Playing sports had strengthened my heart to the point I couldn't be considered a heart patient anymore. That's when I decided to get into the fitness world.

Back then, in the late 1970s, I didn't even know what a gym

was. I was a cheerleader and a country girl. One day I took an aerobics class with a girlfriend. The instructor told me I had rhythm and asked if I'd like to teach a class, so I started teaching aerobics. I fell deeply in love with aerobics, then found the weight room. Soon after, I became a "certified Nautilus instructor"—the closest thing to a present-day "personal trainer" that existed at the time.

I started competing in the Reebok National Aerobic Championship in the late 1980s and early 1990s. I got active in the world of bodybuilding in the 1990's and won many titles. In 1999, I became the women's U.S. Open Tennis champion. Somewhere in there, I got married and had two kids.

My first marriage was already on the rocks when my brother Brian died. When depression was on the verge of overtaking my life, my only relief was through fitness. I would take my aggravation and self-pity out in the gym, and it helped me from going into a deep, dark hole. When I got divorced, I said to myself, "I'm 29, divorced with two kids. How am I going to make a living?" I never once thought what I did as a hobby could be a profession. So I got odd jobs. I waitressed. I sold cars. In 1993, I started my own personal training company, became a certified personal trainer through Colorado State University (CSU) and started Phenomenal Physiques. By 1995, I had saved up enough money that I was able to open my first gym, Bodies by Design. Within five years, one club had grown into a chain.

***

One day in 2000, a man walked into my gym and said, "I want to buy your health clubs." When I asked him why, he replied, "I have done my research and you are going to be my hardest, strongest competition. I want to buy you out."

I was at a crossroads. I asked my mother, "Why would I want to sell my dream?" She said, "Are you only allowed one dream in life?" The thought was a revelation. I took him up on the offer.

From there, I became a consultant and worked with many health clubs all over the U.S. I took an assignment to manage the Teton Sports Club and Spa in Jackson Hole, Wyoming, and kept my personal training business on the side, which allowed me to travel with movie stars and billionaires on the weekend. I was living the high life—private jets to Vegas and Aspen—but I was lonely. I couldn't find true companionship.

So I decided to move back to California, where I worked with Bally Total Fitness. By then I had a reputation as a "fixer," someone who could rescue poorly performing health clubs and turn them around. Jackson Hole had been an 18-month complete turnaround from loss to profitability. Bally offered me a position as a regional district supervisor. This was unheard of at the time. They never hired people off the street—you had to work your way up internally through the organization. I stayed with Bally until 2007. At the same time, I worked as a real estate agent, figuring it was something I could do when my days as a fitness instructor were over. Eventually I turned full-time to the real estate world. Yet even when I made my first million-dollar sale, it never gave me the kick that teaching someone to take control of their life through their body did.

When I moved to Houston I met the man of my dreams—in church, of all places—and re-married at age 47. I was happy. I was living the perfect life, with two fabulous children and two careers. Then, in 2006, Michael died.

***

If God and fitness were my personal cornerstones of resiliency in those dark days, charity work was a huge part of my foundation. I considered my work with Child Legacy International—a nonprofit that provides access to clean water, healthcare and education to children in Africa—part of my legacy to my son. To raise money for CLI, I committed to climb Mt. Kilimanjaro, the largest freestanding mountain in the world.

Before the ascent, my body was infected with a dangerous parasite during a week in Malawi helping drill water wells. Unfortunately I didn't discover the infection until I was 15,000 feet up the mountain. I thought I could fix myself with a little Imodium AD, but over the course of the next 24 hours, I got sicker and sicker. I was suffering from altitude sickness too and extremely dehydrated. Blood was coming from every orifice of my body, and my temperature rocketed to 104 degrees. So I prayed to my son. I needed him to give me my angel wings and help me reach the top. To this day, I'm convinced the only reason I didn't die on Mt. Kilimanjaro was because of Michael. I somehow got to the summit and then back to base camp, where I was carried off on a stretcher. Afterward, a doctor told me there was no reason I made it off that mountain alive.

You don't have to be near death at 19,000 feet for fitness to save your life. A few years into my marriage, my husband Lamar was suddenly feeling listless and had a lot less energy. He had started snoring as well, and I had not married a snorer. One day while playing golf, Lamar couldn't make it back to his cart after a swing. He drove himself to the hospital, where they said he had congestive heart failure. His heart was operating at 25 percent of capacity, with a racing heartbeat of more than 250 beats per minute. Doctors tried giving him medicine. When that failed, they used a pair of defibrillator paddles on his chest to return his heartbeat to a normal rate. My husband was discharged from the hospital with stern instructions: if he wanted to live, he was going to have to strengthen his heart.

I put him on a fitness routine, and we walked miles around our house, twice a day, until we were able to strengthen his heart from 25 percent to 65 percent, just like I had done with my own heart as a child.

***

According to the Department of Health and Human Services, 39.5 percent of adults between the ages of 40 and 59 are obese. From 2003 to 2012, the obesity rate among women aged 60 years and older rose from 31.5 percent to 38.1 percent. Not only that, we're passing our bad habits on to the next generation. The government statistics show that more than one-third of Americans between the ages of 12 and 19 are considered overweight or obese. Rising obesity rates are nothing new, which only makes the phenomenon worse. We've known for years that we're out of shape, and we still aren't doing anything about it!

I've heard all the excuses. Time is scarce, gym memberships can get expensive and it's simply harder to look fit as we get older. My response is always the same: if staying fit was easy, it wouldn't be worth working for! Maintaining our physical health is just like a having a healthy marriage, a fulfilling job, or raising successful children: working hard is not an option.

To change our behavior, we have to change our mindset. There's a popular misconception that our age should dictate how we look. I'm 54 years old, but I've been mistaken for a woman in her 30s. When I became a mother, then a grandmother, I was often told "you don't look like one." That's a nice compliment with a sad implication: older people aren't supposed to look healthy.

My life has shown me that fitness can heal and nurture. It can make you whole, like it did when I lost my brother, and my son, and my biological father—my spiritual rock—as an adult. Now I'm out to prove you don't have to be defined by chronological age or what the world thinks you should feel. I've never accepted the conventional wisdom of doctors and society. At 54, I can still stay in shape and take pride in who I am naked—in body, mind and spirit. Just because society defines you as "middle-aged," that doesn't mean you have to struggle with the same physical, mental and spiritual issues as your peers. You can fight the statistics and win. You can love being naked.

Chapter One

Overview

This diet and exercise program I am sharing with you is one I have used and developed with a team of wellness experts and is also based on years of personal experience. Even though I have been in the fitness and bodybuilding communities for decades, I brought in current experts to make sure I had the most up-to-date and scientific information to share. My team consists of Dr. George Davis, a board certified emergency room doctor and co-owner of a wellness center in Houston; Heather Smith, a licensed nurse practitioner specializing in women's health and wellbeing and Sean Smith, my trainer. Heather and Sean own and operate Sparta Fitness, the gym where I go to work out.

This is a high-protein, low-carb, and vegetable diet with little to no wheat or gluten, or dairy, and also very little sugar. Think of it as *The Scarsdale Diet* of the 21st century, taking into account all the new information we have learned about sugars and gluten over the past three decades.

You should lose somewhere between seven and 20 pounds on this diet and exercise routine, if you stick to it for the 30 days. If you cheat or make too many modifications, your results will be less, but you will still have good results and learn a new way of looking at yourself, food and your relationships with both. It's all up to you.

The meal plans in this book contain approximately 1,400 calories spread over six meals a day (or three meals and three snacks). You can adjust according to your height and weight, but that is the average.

The exercise program is daily, about an hour a day, with specific areas targeted to tone and strengthen your body and reduce your body/fat ratio. You may not lose a lot of pounds, as building muscle replaces fat, but you will lose inches, which is why I have included the measurement chart in Appendix A for you to jot down your progress. I have included mine as well. You can see I started at 174 pounds, with a 14.5 percent of body fat and ended at 162 pounds with nearly 13.9 percent body fat. After three months on the plan, I eventually got down to my goal weight of 155 pounds and eight percent body fat, but that is really for someone who is looking to achieve a high level of fitness. The average woman is fine with 15—25 percent body fat.

I recommend that you work with a personal trainer during this 30-day period, but be warned—a personal trainer is not a babysitter. A personal trainer is someone who is going to take you out of your comfort zone and help you get the results you cannot achieve on your own. However, some of my friends and colleagues who have worked this program have been able to do it without a trainer. There is even a senior citizen who managed to work this program and lose inches and pounds with a much less strenuous version of the plan, so it works for everyone at every level and every age!

It would be irresponsible of me to recommend that you start a diet and exercise routine like this without advising that you meet with your personal physician before going on the diet. You should have your blood analyzed for cholesterol and blood sugars, as well as your hormonal levels.

We all know the basic givens of taking care of yourself, but I will lay them out here as well. Your body will need sleep to repair, recover and rejuvenate, so make sure you get seven or eight hours a night, which most doctors recommend. Make sure you are well hydrated at all times (more on that in my diet). Take a multivitamin. Don't do a strenuous work out on an empty stomach.

And remember to always believe in yourself. Make and follow a plan and you will succeed.

Chapter Two

The Naked in 30 Days Diet

Abs start in the kitchen, not in the gym.

One of the things my trainer, Sean Smith, likes to tell me is to keep it simple. So the NAKED diet is pretty straightforward and easy to follow. Sean provides his clients with The Sparta Diet, similar to the NAKED diet, which is why we see eye to eye and the results speak for themselves.

Over the years, we have learned that a high-protein diet shows the best weight loss, so this diet is exactly that.

In a nutshell, this is a high-protein, low-carb diet that also asks you to avoid alcohol, cow-milk products, processed sugar, wheat, gluten, processed vegetable oils and processed foods and replaces them with seasonal fresh vegetables and fruits, high-quality fats and proteins and non-glutinous grains.

What to Avoid

There are very few absolutes, so we'll start with those.

1) Stick to a grain-free diet

Dr. George says if you eat a grain-free diet, it will eliminate hunger. Recent medical studies have shown that wheat and grains are pro-inflammatory and may be responsible for many of the digestive illnesses we've developed as a nation over the last five decades based on the outdated food pyramids of the 1950s. Wheat and grain products can be easily replaced with alternatives such as almond and coconut flours and blue-corn tortillas.

The reason we remove wheat and gluten from the diet is that the flour and bread of the 21st century is exponentially different from that of your parents and grandparents. Over the decades, agribusiness has created strains of wheat and flour that are impervious to decay, and in doing that have altered their nutrient composition, creating a food product that is misleading, and some believe, even detrimental to your health (Dr. George jokingly refers to them as "Frankenwheat."). We have found that removing wheat and glutens from the diet for 30 days always benefits your health and wellbeing, so we ask you to bear with us on this one (if you want to explore this further, I have included a list of some important resources at the end of this book).

2) Try to cut out cow-milk products.

Dr. George advises women to avoid dairy and other sources of carbohydrates, as they can cause increased water retention. The reason? Metabolically, women who are in their late 30s or early 40s start experiencing peri menopause, which is a slight decrease in their sex hormones estrogen and progesterone. When the balance is tilted in favor of estrogen, they start to gain weight. Add to that the decrease in thyroid hormones, which also causes weight gain and sluggishness, symptoms that often make women feel less comfortable about their bodies and themselves.

So it is just easier to cut out cow milk products altogether for 30 days, especially since there isn't much protein in milk. You can substitute almond milk instead, as well as goat milk.

Again, this is another category of food that has changed dramatically over the decades through chemical and preservative alteration, as well as synthetic hormones that have been added to most cow milk products. In addition, many cheese and yogurts have high fructose corn syrup added, and that complicates digestion.

3) Avoid alcohol

Your body processes alcohol differently than other foods, so it is always recommended that you avoid alcohol when dieting. When alcohol is in your system, it gets processed first and delays the breaking down of foods containing carbohydrates and fat, which are then converted into body fat and stored on your hips and muffin tops.

However, truth be told, I like to have a drink occasionally, and there is no way I am going on a 30-day diet without alcohol for a month. I am a grown woman, after all. So, I choose non-grain alcoholic drinks, which are easier and cleaner to digest. I allow myself an occasional glass of potato vodka on the rocks, with a twist of lime or lemon, because vodka is the cleanest alcohol. Tequila is another non-grain-based alcohol, as it is processed from the agave plant. Wine is also non-grain based but high in sugar, so I opted to remove it from my diet for my 30-day period, but it is permissible, if you must have an occasional drink.

4) Eliminate processed foods.

Eat nothing that comes from a box. Processed foods have had most, if not all, of the nutrients stripped from them and are most likely full of empty calories and chemicals. The fiber necessary to your diet and digestion is also often stripped out of processed foods.

5) Watch your sodium intake.

Everyone knows sodium makes you retain water. We all need some salt in our diets, especially since it is the way we get the mineral iodine, but you have to keep an eye open for store-bought foods. For instance, there is way too much salt and sugar in the average store-bought orange juice. Read the ingredients on your energy or granola bars as well. You'll often find they are loaded with salt and sugars. Unfortunately, if it tastes good, it's usually bad for you.

6) Avoid processed and unnatural sugars.

Anyone on a diet should avoid sugar-filled foods as they are high in calories. Unfortunately, naturally sweetened foods are often slower to digest too, so you have to watch your fruit intake as well. Berries are your best bet. In addition to being high in calories, sugars are also considered empty calories with no real nutritional value. For those reasons, Dr. George recommends that you use the sugar substitute Stevia, which is made from a South American plant, if you must sweeten your food. My trainer Sean suggests you add berries to shakes and meals to sweeten things up.

But be warned, most American store-bought foods have been overrun by the sugar industry, which has put high-fructose corn syrup in everything we eat from bread to juice and even yogurt. Something you think is healthy, may not be.

Needless to say, you'll be avoiding all junk food on this diet, although you can snack on popcorn (without butter), and my trainer recommends a snack of homemade guacamole or salsa and bean chips.

What is on the NAKED in 30 Days Diet?

The NAKED in 30 Days Diet is a high-protein/low-carb/good fat diet that consists of 30 to 50 percent of your calories obtained from protein. The average American diet is comprised of only 10—15 percent protein. This diet also cuts carbohydrate intake considerably by eliminating gluten and replacing it with oats, rice and other non-gluten flours. In order to get a full spectrum of vitamins and minerals, you must also eat a healthy balance of fresh fruits and vegetables and non-gluten grains.

This diet consists of six meals comprised of creative combinations of the following lean proteins, low carbs, fruits and vegetables, oats and rice products. Here is a short list of what you can eat (and I keep it short because you should too; do not confuse yourself by adding):

Poultry

Lean turkey (skinless breasts or tenderloin)
Lean chicken (skinless)
Lean ground turkey
Turkey cutlets
Eggs (yolk is good fat, white is where the protein is)

Beef

Lean cuts of beef (such as brisket, flank steak)
Eye of round roast or steak
Sirloin tip side steak
Top or bottom round roast
Top sirloin steak

Seafood

Cod (wild)
Salmon
MahiMahi
Yellowfin tuna
Tuna
Tilapia (out of China, if possible)
Snapper
Orange roughy
Halibut

<u>NAKED Tip</u>

Not all seafood items are great for your diet. As Sean Smith of Sparta Fitness says, "Shrimp and lobster, for example, have very few nutritional benefits." Be careful not to veer from the seafood items listed above as they have been specifically chosen.

Nuts

Raw or roasted almonds
Cashews
Walnuts
Pecans
Peanuts
Pine nuts

<u>NAKED Tip</u>

The USDA defines an extra-lean cut of beef as a 3.5-ounce serving (about 100 grams) that contains less than five grams total fat, two grams saturated fat, and 95 milligrams cholesterol

<u>NAKED Tip</u>

Three ounces of meat is about the size of a deck of cards, so six ounces is twice that.

Greens

Romaine
Green leaf
Spinach
Arugula
Swiss chard
Kale

NAKED Tip

The darker the leafy green, the better, thus spinach is a great option if you like the taste. I like a mix of baby spinach and baby kale. The darker leafy greens contain the most nutrients, vitamins and minerals. They also contain chlorophyll, which is great for your blood, and fiber, great for a healthy colon! Many greens, such as kale, collard greens and arugula, also contain some cancer-preventing compounds called isothiocyanates and indoles that occur naturally in certain vegetables.

Vegetables

Avocado
Cauliflower
Asparagus
Celery
Zucchini
Brussels sprouts
Eggplant
Green and red peppers
Tomatoes
Peas
Spinach
Mushrooms
Onions
Garlic
Olives
Capers
Scallions
Peppers
Herbs

Toppings & Spreads

Raw or organic peanut butter
Raw or organic almond butter
Hummus
Condiments such as catsup and mustard (but no mayonnaise)

Fruits & Berries

Generally speaking, fruits help fight inflammation because they are low in calories and fat, yet high in antioxidants. The more fibrous berries are the best for you, help you feel fuller longer, and have many additional do-good properties. But some fruits, such as bananas, are high in sugar and should be minimized or avoided entirely, thus I have not included the higher-sugar fruits in this list.

Raspberries
Blackberries
Blueberries
Strawberries
Green apples
Oranges
Grapefruits
Melon
Grapes
Pears
Lemons
Limes

Carbohydrates & Other Proteins

Whey protein supplement (many flavors)
Vegan protein powder like Garden of Life Raw Fit protein powder
Oats and oatmeal
Cream of rice
Rice cakes
Beans
Popcorn

Beverages

Juices
Coffee
Tea

Sweeteners & Seasonings

Stevia
Truvia
Herbs
Spices

Dressings

Vinaigrette dressing
Virgin olive oil
Balsamic vinegar
Apple cider vinegar

Use this as a basic shopping list, although you can look up the recommended shopping list put together by Dr. Oz and add items, as long as you stay away from the gluten and starches.

This book doesn't contain complex recipes because the meals are so simple to prepare and very basic. They are all pretty much mix and match, rinse and repeat over 30 days.

Of course, all your food should be grilled, baked, boiled or broiled.

If you must use a cooking base, you can use olive oil, but I prefer coconut oil. I cook my eggs in it. You can also cook with chicken broth.

My trainer recommends that I add a tablespoon of Udos oil to my daily meal plan instead of a fish oil, which can cause belching. Udos is a natural dietary supplement of blended plant oils of a two to one ratio of Omega-3 and Omega-6 fatty acids (the good fats), which is considered the right combination for a healthy nutritional balance. The one requirement is that you have to keep it refrigerated at all times. It comes in gel caps, but they can go bad quickly. You can buy it in a health food store or online.

There are also some basic guidelines you need to be very mindful of when you are on any diet, but especially one that changes what you would normally eat.

Always make sure you are well hydrated. My trainer, Sean, says, "Take your body weight and divide it by two and apply that number to ounces, so if you are 150 pounds, half of that is 75, so drink 75 ounces of water daily. This is a bit over nine cups." I drink about a gallon of water a day because, as Sean explains, high amounts of protein can be hard on the kidneys. "The increased protein can make you dehydrated if you don't flush it out. The water helps to process the proteins through the kidneys."

Lack of water can lead to dehydration, which can be a dangerous condition that can drain your energy, which can be especially debilitating when you are dieting and exercising. Dehydration occurs when you don't have enough water in your body to optimally process normal bodily functions.

The human body is comprised of mostly water, which makes up 60 percent of your body weight. Without water, every system in your body would be unable to function. Water flushes toxins out of all your organs and carries nutrients to your cells.

Imagine your body as a sewer system. You need to flush out the waste. You need to stay hydrated for brain function and to push the sewage through your system. The faster you can push the fluids out, the faster you get better. Skin, hair, nail, brain and cell growth all need hydration. Most cravings are the result of thirst.

I keep a bottle of water with me in the car and in my gym bag, as well as in my pocketbook at all times. I make sure I have water when I leave the house along with my phone, my wallet and my keys.

Throughout my adult life, I have learned that the best way to keep focused is to plan, so I plan ahead when I am going on a diet. I would recommend you shop for a number of the foods on this list before you begin the diet so you can never use the excuse of not having variety or ingredients to go off the diet.

I travel a lot for business and charity, and I know when I am going to be away from my comfort zone. While I know I can always order a salad, or a simple serving of tuna or salmon or chicken breast in a restaurant, I often travel with packets of rice crackers and tuna, or rice cakes, so I am never starving and stranded. There's even natural singles of peanut butter you can buy for travel.

A lot of people use food as energy because they are really tired, but if you eat right, and get enough sleep, you will be a well-oiled machine.

Most people live to eat. If people would eat to live, they would live differently. If you can eat to live, you will only eat what your body needs to survive.

Chapter Three

Exercise

This 30-day workout plan consists of many different types of resistance and cardiovascular training exercises. It is good to change up your workout routine often so you do not reach a plateau.

In this 30-day plan, we suggest using a combination of resistance training with weights, bands and machines, high intensity interval training (HIIT) cardio, and weight training. All of these methods combined with a clean diet are a great way to burn fat while sustaining muscle.

Your cardiovascular exercise is as critical as the weight training. Cardiovascular exercise is any movement that increases your heart rate and blood circulation. Because your heart has to work much harder during exercise and pumps blood around your body at a much faster rate, the cardiovascular exercise allows your body to become better and more efficient at pumping blood. When everyday activities, such as climbing stairs, lifting heavy objects or running around in the yard with your kids become easier, this means you are doing a good job with your cardio exercises. Over time, your heart rate will slow down during cardio exercises since your heart will have gotten better at moving blood through your body—and that's the goal, to increase the cardio while lowering the heart rate during cardiovascular exercise.

You can find all of the exercises in this book on my YouTube page https://www.youtube.com/user/theresaroemer. However, in order to ensure proper technique, which is crucial when executing an exercise, I will also be describing them in this chapter.

This is a 30-day program to transform your body by losing fat and maintaining or building lean muscle. Therefore, there will only be one rest day, but use the rest day wisely and stretch or take stairs wherever possible.

Working out gives you energy because it releases endorphins, which gives you a sense of wellbeing, or a natural high or rush. I find if I work out early, it sets the mood for the entire day. If I can work out in the morning, there is a huge difference in my personality and energy level.

My workout begins around 8:00 a.m. and my home gym has just about everything I need in it: treadmill, elliptical trainer, weights, benches, ropes, resistance tubing, weighted bars, balance boards and rubber balls, just to name a few pieces of my equipment. However, all you really need is a mat, a pair of weights (from two to five pounds, depending on your comfort level), a resistance ball and some resistance bands to get a good home workout. You don't need fancy workout clothes or matching attire, but, of course, it's nice to have and will make you feel good. Make sure what you are wearing is comfortable so it doesn't impede your rapid movement. The right sneakers or gym shoes are critical, as they must provide your feet with good support. Your feet take a beating when you're working out a lot and heartily, and those sneakers are their cushion. Ladies, you also need a good support bra. Take your time making this purchase and try a few to discover the right make and model for *the girls*.

I aim for three days of cardio and three days of weight training every week with one day of rest. Rest in my case is a relative term because my home is filled with stairs that I climb three or four times a day, happily and intentionally, to make sure I am using my legs and glutes as much as possible.

My workouts are typically comprised of three to four exercises per body part, three to four sets at a time with 20 reps each, alternating with cardio every other day. I work on my abs daily because this is the one area of muscles you can train every day and not over-train, and an area that usually could use the extra work out on a woman's body.

A woman's body is greatly affected by her hormone levels, especially as she ages. While this is also true for men, it is much more obvious to the naked eye on a woman's body, as the shape of her upper arms and waist are due to estrogen levels. This is why the backs of the arms and the midriff are such problem areas as women age and go through menopause.

Below is my typical workout schedule:

Day 1—One hour of cardio
Day 2—Upper body strength training
Day 3—One hour of cardio
Day 4—Legs and glutes
Day 5—One hour of cardio
Day 6—Chest, back and shoulders
Day 7—Rest or stretch

Here is a description of each workout:

Warm-Up Stretches

Shoulder and Arm Warm-Up

You will need a six-foot rod for this exercise. The pole from a broom will do.

Stand with the rod in front of you, bring it over the top of your head and behind your back. Bring it back over the top of your head and back to the start position in front of you. Perform this exercise for approximately three minutes to warm up the upper body before any upper-body workout. Repeat circuit three to five times. Rest period 30—45 seconds

Hamstring Glute Stretch

Lying flat on your back, bring one leg up straight and make a figure four with the opposite leg. Reach your arms up to grab the upwardly extended leg at the calf or at the thigh (never pull at the knee) and pull toward your chest. You should feel a nice stretch in your hip muscles, including the glutes and piriformis muscle. This is also a great stretch to relieve back pain. Repeat one rep on each side.

Lower Back Stretch

Lie flat on your back with your legs extended. Bring one leg up, bent at a 90 degree angle. Use the opposite arm to gently pull the knee so the bent leg moves across the body. The corresponding arm to the leg should be stretched straight out (e.g. if you are bringing your right leg over to the left side, your right arm is straight out to the right.). This provides a nice stretch in your glutes and core. Repeat on the opposite side.

Abs

Abdominal Crossover

On an exercise mat in a lying-down position, bend one knee and place your ankle on the opposite straight leg at the knee. Place your hand behind your head on the same side of your body that the knee is bent. Take the opposite arm and place out to your side at shoulder height. Take that extended arm and crunch up, crossing that straight arm over and out past the bent knee. Repeat 15 times on each side for three sets.

Ab Rollers

Kneeling on a mat, position your hands on the ab wheel and roll your upper body out in front of you, extending to an almost straight position, and then pull yourself back into your starting position. Caution: only go out as far as you feel comfortable so you don't strain your lower back. Baby steps are a good way to start out on this exercise. Three sets of 20 reps.

Lower Ab Crunches

Lying on a mat with your legs in the air and crossed, place your arms down at your sides or partially tucked under your bottom. Using your abs, lift your bottom slightly off the floor and release, allowing your bottom to land back on the floor. The key here is to use your abs and not your legs to get your bottom up off the floor. This is a lower abdominal crunch. Do three sets of 20 reps.

Resistance Ball Crunches

Lying on a resistance ball with knees bent and only your lower back on the ball, place your arms behind your head with your elbows out to the side and slowly crunch your abs by slightly raising your shoulders. Lower yourself back down and repeat the motion for three sets of 25 reps. Remember to exhale as you crunch.

Straight-Legged Ab Crunches

Position yourself on a mat lying flat on your back with your legs straight and your hands behind your ears, with your elbows bent. Raise your shoulders off the mat, keeping your elbows out to the side and chin tucked into your chest. You should exhale as you crunch your abs during this exercise. Repeat 25 reps for three sets. Remember not to pull on your head when raising yourself up, as it can cause neck strain. You want your abs to be doing all the work.

If you find this is too difficult on your back, you might want to try it with your knees bent.

Straight-Leg Flutters

Lie on your back with your legs together and extended out straight. Place your arms out to the sides of your body with your palms down, or you can put your hands under your butt.

Placing your hands under your butt does two things. First, it positions your hips and pelvis up just a little bit, which helps in keeping your feet elevated. Second, it takes strain off your lower back. If you choose to have your hands out to the sides of your body, concentrate on keeping your lower back pressed to the floor. Contract your abs and keep them tight throughout the exercise. Lift your legs off the ground about six inches. Lift your head and shoulders slightly off the ground. This will bring your upper abs into the exercise. Now start flutter kicking. Raise one leg up a few inches and bring it back to the starting position. While it's on its way down, raise the other leg. This is a timed 30-second exercise consisting of three reps.

V-Ups

Lying on a mat with your legs stretched outward and your arms stretched overhead, bring your arms up and legs up at the same time to form a V with your body. Legs are lifted almost straight up and arms are brought up to meet the legs, slightly bringing your shoulders off the mat to touch the legs. Repeat this motion for three sets of 20 reps. This is a variation on sit-ups. They are hard but very effective.

Back

Assisted Back Pull-Ups

On an assisted pull-up machine, gasp the top bar with your hands shoulder width apart. Make sure you loaded enough weight on the stack to help assist you in your pull-ups. If the pull-ups are too hard, add more weight. You want the pull-ups to be hard but not impossible. As you get better at this, you will be able to take more weight off and hopefully one day do pull-ups with no assistance at all. Step onto the assist bar and let it lower to the floor. Using your back muscles, pull yourself up, all the while squeezing your lower body. Do three sets of 15 reps. There is no better exercise than the pull-up to establish a beautiful V-shaped back.

Lat Pull-Downs

Sit on a bench with arms extended above your head shoulder width apart and hanging onto a cable machine bar with 50 lbs. Keeping your back straight, pull the bar down to slightly under the chin and raise the bar back up to starting position. The key here is to use your back muscles, not your arm muscles, so you need to focus on squeezing your back as you pull down the bar. Do three sets of 15 reps.

One-Arm Dumbbell Rows

Choose a flat bench and place a dumbbell on either side of it. Place the right leg on top of the end of the bench, bend your torso forward from the waist until your upper body is parallel to the floor, and place your right hand on the other end of the bench for support. Use the left hand to pick up the dumbbell on the floor and hold the weight while keeping your lower back straight. The palm of the hand should be facing your torso. Pull the resistance straight up to the side of your chest, keeping your upper arm close to your side and keeping the torso stationary. Concentrate on squeezing the back muscles once you reach the full contracted position. Also, make sure the force is performed with the back muscles and not the arms. Finally, the upper torso should remain stationary and only the arms should move. The forearms should do no other work except for holding the dumbbell; therefore, do not try to pull the dumbbell up using the forearms.

Lower the resistance straight down to the starting position. Repeat the movement 15 times on each side. Switch sides and repeat again with the other arm.

Seated Cable Rows

On a chest press machine, sit down facing the seat with your chest pressed up against the back of the seat. Extend your arms grasping the handles and pull the handles with 50 pounds back toward your armpits, squeezing the middle of your back as you pull back. Move handles back to staring position and repeat motion again. Do three sets of 15 reps.

Speed Rows

When performing a speed row with resistance bands, begin by selecting your desired resistance. Hold a handle in each hand and keep your feet straight and flat on the floor. Next, hold the handles out in front of you with your elbows extended. In one explosive motion, row back by bringing your thumbs toward your armpits and squeezing your shoulder blades together. Be sure not to shrug your shoulders or jut your head forward. Repeat this as fast as possible, with control, for the desired number of repetitions. This is a timed 30-second exercise consisting of three reps.

Arms

Barbell 21's

Stand upright and grab a barbell with an underhand grip. Place your hands shoulder width apart and allow your arms to hang toward the floor. Tuck your elbows tight to the sides of your body. Curl upward until you make a 90-degree angle at your elbow. Relax your arms back to full extension and repeat six more curls reaching the 90-degree angle at your elbow. From this position, curl the weight up until the barbell is one to two inches away from your shoulder. Lower the weight back to the 90-degree-elbow position and repeat six more times. Now, allow your arms to return to full extension. This time, curl your arms from full extension all the way to full extension. Keep curling until the bar is about one to two inches away from your shoulder. Repeat six more curls through this full range of motion to complete a total of 21 curls.

Alternating Bicep Curls

Standing with your feet shoulder width apart and ten-pound dumbbells in your hands hanging down to your side, slowly bring one arm up bending at the elbow and bring the dumbbell to shoulder squeezing your bicep. Release and bring arm back down into starting position. Repeat motion with opposite arm. This is an exercise with arms alternating the movement. Do three sets of 15 reps each arm. This exercise can also be done sitting on a bench or chair for more back support.

Hammer Curls

Stand up with your torso upright and a dumbbell in each hand being held at arm's length. The elbows should be close to the torso. The palms should be facing your torso. This will be your starting position. Now, while holding your upper arm stationary, exhale and curl the weight forward while contracting the biceps. Continue to raise the weight until the biceps are fully contracted and the dumbbell is at shoulder level. Hold the contracted position for a brief moment as you squeeze the biceps. Tip: focus on keeping the elbow stationary and only moving your forearm. After the brief pause, inhale and slowly begin the lower the dumbbells back to the starting position. Do 15 reps per arm.

Seated Concentration One-Arm Bicep Curls

Sit on a bench or chair grasping a ten-pound dumbbell in one hand, with your elbow resting against your knee with your opposite hand placed on your opposite knee for support. Lower the weight to the floor. Curl the same arm back up toward your opposite shoulder while keeping your back straight. Repeat 15 times and then switch arms and position. Repeat for three sets of 15 reps with each arm.

Seated Bicep Dumbbell Curls

Sitting on an inclined 45-degree bench with eight-pound dumbbells in your hands, hang your arms down to your sides. Slowly curl the weights up toward your shoulders and lower them back down to starting position. Repeat movement 15 reps for three sets.

Standing Barbell Curls

In a standing position with a 20-pound weighted bar with hands shoulder width apart, start with elbows tucked into ribs and bar out in front. Lower the bar to your legs and bring it back up to the starting position out in front. Repeat this movement for three sets of 15 reps.

Standing Bicep Curls

Stand up with your torso upright while holding a cable curl bar that is attached to a low pulley. Grab the cable bar with your hands shoulder width apart and keep the elbows close to the torso. Your palms should be facing up (supinated grip). This will be your starting position. While holding the upper arms stationary, curl the weights while contracting the biceps as you breathe out. Only the forearms should move. Continue the movement until your biceps are fully contracted and the bar is at shoulder level. Hold the contracted position for a second as you squeeze the muscle. Slowly begin to bring the curl bar back to starting position as your breathe in. Repeat.

Twisting Curls

Grab a pair of dumbbells and let them hang at arm's length at your sides. Stand upright with a tight torso. Your palms should be facing your body. Slowly curl one arm up to the shoulder. Midway through the curl, rotate the wrist so it faces your body at the top of the movement. Pause for a second and slowly return the dumbbell to the starting position, rotating back midway through the movement. Alternate arms. Be sure to utilize a full range of motion where you begin in full extension and reach peak contraction. Keep the elbows stationary throughout the entire movement. Perform the movement with a controlled pace, not allowing momentum to contribute.

Tricep Dips

Sit on a bench or chair and put your hands next to you with your hands facing out toward your legs. Put your legs on a bench across from you or put your feet flat on the floor, bent at the knee. Drop your butt off the bench down toward the floor and, using your arms to push your body weight back up, straighten your arms. Do three sets of 15 reps.

Tricep High Lateral Rope Pull-Downs

Standing at the cable machine with 30 pounds and rope attached, place hands at the bottom of the ropes with your elbows tucked in close to your ribs. Pull the rope down toward the ground, keeping your elbows tucked in. Squeeze your triceps at the bottom and bring the rope back up to the starting position. Do three sets of 15—20 reps.

Tricep Kickbacks

Bend over a bench or chair, resting your inside knee and inside arm on the bench or chair. Straighten your outside leg and position it farther back to get your back flat like a table top. Take your outside arm with a five-pound weight (or your desired weight) and tuck your elbow into your side holding the weight down (your arm will resemble a pendulum on a clock). Now kick your hand with the weight in it back toward your hip. Do three sets of 15 reps per arm.

Tricep Overhead Press

Sitting or standing, take a ten-pound dumbbell (or your desired weight) and grasp one end of the dumbbell with both hands and keep your elbows close to your head. Lower your hands with the dumbbell behind your head and press back up toward the ceiling. Do three sets of 15 reps.

Tricep Push-downs

Attach a straight or angled bar to a high pulley and grab with an overhand grip (palms facing down) at shoulder width. Standing upright with the torso straight and a very small inclination forward, bring the upper arms close to your body and perpendicular to the floor. The forearms should be pointing up toward the pulley as they hold the bar. This is your starting position. Using the triceps, bring the bar down until it touches the front of your thighs and the arms are fully extended perpendicular to the floor. The upper arms should always remain stationary next to your torso and only the forearms should move. Exhale as you perform this movement. After a second hold at the contracted position, bring the bar slowly up to the starting point. Breathe in as you perform this step. Repeat for the recommended amount of repetitions.

Tricep Stretch

In a sitting or standing position, reach one hand back behind your head and use the opposite hand to gently grasp the elbow of the arm that is extended behind the head. Do once on each side, holding for 10—20 seconds.

Legs

Alternating Jumping Lunges

Start in a split-stance position with your hands on your hips, your torso upright, and your knees about bent at a 90-degree angle. Push your chest out and lower your rear knee toward the ground in a lunge while keeping your front shin as vertical as possible. Push explosively off the ground, jumping and switching the position of your legs while in mid air, landing into the lunge position with the opposite leg forward. Repeat, switching legs on each jump. Avoid landing too hard. Land on the ground as softly as possible. Make sure to use a full range of motion. Lower yourself until your back knee lightly grazes the ground. Avoid bending the torso forward. Keep your chest tall and upright the entire time. Make sure to keep the torso from rotating. Keep your chest square to the wall in front of you.

Anterior Reach Lunge

Start standing with your feet together. Beginners should start with bodyweight while more advanced lifters can hold weights by their sides. Intermediate lifters or people suffering from low back pain may want to do the lunge with a front reach instead of adding weight. Step forward with one foot. Beginners can keep the step forward smaller. A bigger step forward will make the move more difficult. Step forward and bend the front knee slightly as you hinge over. All of your weight should basically be in your front leg with your back leg used for balance and support. While you are stepping forward, your weight shouldn't continue to go forward as you hinge over. Your front heel should be firmly on the ground while your back leg stays straight. Your back should also be flat as you lean/hinge over. The more you lean over, the harder the move. *Do not move your back toward the ground.* It doesn't matter if the weights touch the ground or if you can only lean over a little bit. It only matters that you push the butt back, keep the core engaged and the back flat as you hinge over. If you do the reach instead of holding weights, you will reach your hands overhead and in front of you as you hinge over. Do not round your back as you reach. Feel a nice stretch in your glute and hamstring as you hinge over. Make sure your weight isn't going forward into your front toe. The heel of the front foot should be firmly planted on the ground. After you hinge over, stand up and step back. You can choose to complete all reps on one side or alternate legs as you go.

Leg Extensions

For this exercise you will need to use a leg extension machine. First choose your weight and sit on the machine with your legs under the pad (feet pointed forward) and your hands holding the side bars. This will be your starting position. Tip: you will need to adjust the pad so it falls on top of your lower leg (just above your feet). Also, make sure your legs form a 90-degree angle between the lower and upper leg. If the angle is less than 90 degrees, that means the knee is over the toes which in turn creates undue stress at the knee joint. If the machine is designed that way, either look for another machine or just make sure that when you start executing the exercise you stop going down once you hit the 90-degree angle. Using your quadriceps, extend your legs to the maximum as you exhale. Ensure that the rest of the body remains stationary on the seat. Pause a second on the contracted position. Slowly lower the weight back to the original position as you inhale, ensuring that you do not go past the 90-degree angle limit. Repeat for the recommended amount of times.

Leg Squats

This exercise can be done in a variety of ways using a squat rack, dumbbells or a resistance exercise ball. No matter which way you choose to do it, the proper way to do this exercise is still the same. If you choose the squat rack, position yourself with the weighted bar across the top of your back resting across your shoulders. With your legs shoulder width apart, release the weighted bar of 25 pounds or desired weight and bend your knees down into a sitting position, pressing your back into the weighted bar for stability and no risk of straining your back. Squeeze your glutes and legs to press yourself back up into a standing position again. Repeat for three sets of 15—20 reps.

If using dumbbells, place the ten-pound dumbbells in each hand resting them on your shoulders and repeat the same motion of exercise. If using a resistance exercise ball, place the ball behind your lower back, resting it up against a wall. Repeat the same sitting motion, pressing your body against the ball as it rolls up and down the wall.

Lying Glute Bridge/Hamstring and Glute Workout

Lie on a mat with one foot on the workout ball and aim the other foot toward the ceiling, elevating your pelvis off the floor. Drop your pelvis back down to the floor while keeping one foot pointing toward the ceiling and the other foot on the workout ball. Repeat this exercise doing 20 reps and then switch feet. Do three sets of 20 reps per leg.

Lying Leg Hamstring Curls

Lie on a mat with an exercise ball under your heels. Lift your pelvis off the floor and roll the ball toward your butt. Roll the ball back out while keeping your butt elevated. Repeat this exercise. Perform three sets of 20 reps.

Jump Squats

Cross your arms over your chest. With your head up and your back straight, position your feet shoulder width apart. Keeping your back straight and chest up, squat as you inhale until your upper thighs are parallel, or lower, to the floor. Now pressing mainly with the ball of your feet, jump straight up as high as possible, using the thighs like springs. Exhale during this portion of the movement. When you touch the floor again, immediately squat down and jump again. Repeat for the recommended amount of repetitions.

Leg Press

Using a leg press machine, sit down on the machine and place your legs on the platform directly in front of you at a medium (shoulder width) foot stance. (Note: for the purposes of this discussion, we will use the medium stance described above, which targets overall development; however you can choose any of the three stances described in the foot-positioning section). Lower the safety bars holding the weighted platform in place and press the platform all the way up until your legs are fully extended in front of you. Tip: make sure you do not lock your knees. Your torso and legs should make a perfect 90-degree angle. This will be your starting position. As you inhale, slowly lower the platform until your upper and lower legs make a 90-degree angle. Pushing mainly with your heels and using your quadriceps, go back to the starting position as you exhale. Repeat for the recommended amount of repetitions and be sure to lock the safety pins properly once you are done. You do not want that platform falling on you fully loaded.

Smith Machine Squats

To begin, first set the bar on the height that best matches your height. Once the correct height is chosen and the bar is loaded, step under the bar and place the back of your shoulders (slightly below the neck) across it. Hold on to the bar using both arms at each side (palms facing forward), unlock it and lift it off the rack by first pushing with your legs and at the same time straightening your torso. Position your legs using a shoulder-width, medium stance with the toes slightly pointed out. Keep your head up at all times and also maintain a straight back. This will be your starting position. Begin to slowly lower the bar by bending the knees as you maintain a straight posture with the head up. Continue down until the angle between the upper leg and the calves becomes slightly less than 90 degrees (the point at which the upper legs are below parallel to the floor). Inhale as you perform this portion of the movement. Begin to raise the bar as you exhale by pushing the floor with your heel as you straighten your legs again and go back to the starting position.

Sideways Duck Squats

Stand next to a bar that is set at slightly higher than waist level. Step sideways as you push your hips back and bring your torso toward the floor to duck under the bar. Stand up on the other side of the bar and prepare to repeat back and forth. Focus on keeping your chest up and your back flat. Keep your weight in your heels at all times. Avoid rounding your back throughout the movement.

Standing Lunges

In a standing position with a weighted ten-pound exercise ball, lunge forward with one leg, holding the weighted ball out in front of you. The front bent knee should not be positioned past the foot.

Remember, the bent knee should be directly over the foot to avoid injury. Bring that bent leg back to standing position and lower the ball. Repeat the same move with your opposite leg, raising the weighted ball out in front of you as you lunge forward again. Do a total of 15 reps with each leg for three sets.

Step-Ups

Stand up straight while holding a dumbbell in each hand (palms facing the sides of your legs). Place the right foot on the elevated platform. Step on the platform by extending the hip and the knee of your right leg. Use the heel mainly to lift the rest of your body up and place the foot of the left leg on the platform as well. Breathe out as you execute the force required to come up. Step down with the left leg by flexing the hip and knee of the right leg as you inhale. Return to the original standing position by placing the right foot next to the left foot on the initial position. Repeat with the right leg, then the left leg, for three reps of 30 seconds each.

Straight-Legged Dead Lift

Stand with your legs shoulder width apart with a 20-pound (or desired) weighted bar. Bend over at the waist, lowering the weight toward the floor, keeping your back flat. You should feel the stretch in your hamstrings, squeezing your glutes, then bring your body back up to a standing position. Repeat exercise for three sets of 15 reps. This exercise should be felt in your hamstrings and glutes.

Walking Lunges

Stand upright, feet together, and take a controlled step forward with your right leg, lowering your hips toward the floor by bending both knees at 90-degree angles. The back knee should point toward but not touch the ground, and your front knee should be directly over the ankle. Press your right heel into the ground and push off with your left foot to bring your left leg forward, stepping with control into a lunge on the other side. This completes two reps. Do three sets of 20 reps each.

Shoulders

Seated Dumbbell Press

Sitting on a bench or chair, bring your arms up to the outsides of your shoulders with ten-pound dumbbells (or desired weight) in each hand. In this starting position, press the dumbbells straight up over your head toward the ceiling. Bring back down to your starting position and repeat. Your arms should be in the position of a field goal on a football field when in your starting position. Do three sets of 15 reps.

Shoulder Rope Swings

Wrap weighted ropes around something sturdy and lay them out in front of you. Standing with legs shoulder width apart, grasp the ends of the ropes and raise your arms up and down in a flutter motion for a timed session of 30 seconds. Rest for one minute and repeat for another 30 seconds. Do three sets of 30 seconds.

Weighted Ball Toss

You will need a partner for this exercise. Lacking one, this movement can be performed against a wall. Begin facing your partner holding a medicine ball at your torso with both hands. Pull the ball to your chest and reverse the motion by extending through the elbows. For sports applications, you can take a step as you throw. Your partner should catch the ball and throw it back to you. Receive the throw with both hands at chest height. This is a timed exercise. Do three sets of 30 reps.

Side Lateral Seated Dumbbell Raises

Sit on a bench or chair holding eight-pound dumbbells in each hand with them down to your sides. Slowly raise them out to the side to shoulder height. Lower them back down and repeat the exercise for three sets of 15 reps. Remember to try to keep your elbows up during the motion.

Dumbbell Front Raises

Pick a couple of dumbbells and stand with a straight torso and the dumbbells in front of your thighs at arm's length with your palms facing your thighs. This will be your starting position. While maintaining the torso stationary (no swinging), lift the left dumbbell to the front with a slight bend in the elbow and the palms always facing down. Continue to go up until your arm is slightly above parallel to the floor. Exhale as you execute this portion of the movement and pause for a second at the top. Inhale after the second pause. Now lower the dumbbell slowly to the starting position as you simultaneously lift the right dumbbell. Continue alternating in this fashion for three sets of 15 reps on each arm.

Dumbbell Upright Rows

Grasp a dumbbell in each hand with a pronated (palms forward) grip with your hands slightly less than shoulder width. The dumbbells should be resting on top of your thighs. Your arms should be extended with a slight bend at the elbows and your back should be straight. This will be your starting position. Use your side shoulders to lift the dumbbells as you exhale. The dumbbells should be close to the body as you move them up, and the elbows should drive the motion. Continue to lift them until they nearly touch your chin. Tip: your elbows should drive the motion. As you lift the dumbbells, your elbows should always be higher than your forearms. Also, keep your torso stationary and pause for a second at the top of the movement. Lower the dumbbells back slowly to the starting position. Inhale as you perform this portion of the movement. Repeat for the recommended amount of repetitions.

Be very careful with how much weight you use in this exercise. Too much weight leads to bad form, which in turn can cause shoulder injury. I've seen this too many times, so please no jerking, swinging and cheating. Also, if you suffer from shoulder problems, you may want to stay away from upright rows and substitute some form of lateral raises.

Chest

Standard Push-Ups

Start with your palms flat on the ground and extend your legs behind you so your weight is on your toes. Make sure your body is in a straight line from your neck to your ankles. Position your hands so your wrists are stacked directly below your shoulders. Lower your body by bending your elbows, keeping your body rigid and moving it as one unit. Lower until your upper arms are about parallel to the ground, then press back up, straightening your elbows. Do three sets of 15 reps.

Dumbbell Presses

Lie down on a flat bench with a dumbbell in each hand resting on top of your thighs. Your palms will be facing each other. Then, using your thighs to help raise the dumbbells, lift the dumbbells one at a time so you can hold them in front of you at shoulder width apart. Once at shoulder width, rotate your wrists forward so your palms are facing away from you. The dumbbells should be just to the sides of your chest, with your upper arm and forearm creating a 90-degree angle. Be sure to maintain full control of the dumbbells at all times. This will be your starting position. Then, as you breathe out, use your chest to push the dumbbells up. Lock your arms at the top of the lift and squeeze your chest, hold for a second and then begin coming down slowly. Tip: ideally, lowering the weight should take about twice as long as raising it. Repeat the movement for three sets of 15 reps of your training program. When you are done, do not drop the dumbbells next to you as this is dangerous to your rotator cuffs in your shoulders and others working out around you. Just lift your legs from the floor, bending at the knees, twist your wrists so your palms are facing each other and place the dumbbells on top of your thighs. When both dumbbells are touching your thighs, simultaneously push your upper torso up (while pressing the dumbbells against your thighs) and also perform a slight kick forward with your legs (keeping the dumbbells on top of the thighs). By doing this combined movement, the momentum will help you get back to a sitting position with both dumbbells still on top of your thighs. At this moment you can place the dumbbells on the floor.

Reverse Push-Ups on the Rubber Ball

Standing behind the resistance ball, crouch and place your abdominals on top of the ball. Roll forward until your hands reach the floor in front of the ball. Walk your hands out until only your feet remain on top of the ball. Contract the core and hold a strong link—

your body should be in a straight and firm line from feet to head. As you bend at the elbows to lower your chest to the floor, maintain your balance on the ball. Keep your torso facing square to the floor.

Advanced version: In the push-up position, lift one foot off the ball and work to balance as you lower and push up. Keep hips and shoulders in alignment. Do three reps of 15 sets.

Below are some additional core training exercises my trainer often adds to my routine, for 20—30 minutes of core training:

Bosu Ball Spiderman Planks

In a high or low plank position, alternate bringing each knee to the outside of your elbow on the same side. Do one to 15 reps per side.

Bicycle Crunches

Lie flat on the floor with your lower back pressed to the ground. For this exercise, you will need to put your hands beside your head. Be careful, however, not to strain with the neck as you perform it. Now lift your shoulders into the crunch position. Bring knees up to where they are perpendicular to the floor, with your lower legs parallel to the floor. This will be your starting position. Now simultaneously, slowly go through a cycle pedal motion, kicking forward with the right leg and bringing in the knee of the left leg. Bring your right elbow close to your left knee by crunching to the side as you breathe out. Go back to the initial position as you breathe in. Crunch to the opposite side as you cycle your legs and bring your left elbow closer to your right knee and exhale. Continue alternating in this manner until all of the recommended repetitions for each side have been completed. Do ten to 15 reps per side.

Bosu Ball Side Planks

Rest your right forearm on top of the dome, stack your left foot on top of your right and lift your body off the ground. Make sure you're in a straight line from head to feet. Contract your abs and squeeze your glutes. Hold for 30 seconds, then switch sides. Do 10—15 reps per side.

Suspended Mountain Climbers

Sit on the floor facing suspension trainer loops in low position. Place your right foot in left lower loop. Cross your left leg over your right leg placed in the right lower loop. Turn your body to right and place your hands on floor, shoulder width apart. Turn your body to kneel on hands and knees. Reposition your hands (shoulder width or slightly wider) at desired distance from suspension trainer so your body is square with suspension trainer straps. With arms straight, raise your knees from the ground so your body is supported by your arms and the suspension trainer. Bend one leg so your knee is pointing down while keeping the other leg extended out straight. Simultaneously alternate leg positions by straightening the bent leg behind, while bending the straight leg forward. Repeat a total of three to six sets for 30—45 seconds.

As I mentioned earlier, it is essential that women work their abdominal muscles—any day and every day. These include combinations of standing, sitting and floor exercises (such as crunches, reverse crunches, side oblique crunches, hanging knee lifts), and these muscles cannot be over-trained.

The most important thing I have learned from years as a professional in fitness is that you must listen to your body, and that each person's body is different. This is critical because so many of us compare ourselves to others who are younger or fitter or professional entertainers, and that is dangerous. We simply are not all built the same. Comparisons will get you into trouble. If your body tells you to take it easy, do it. If you know you need to push yourself, do that instead. Some days I really kick my own butt, and like all of us, I have days where I want to be lazy too. You must never feel guilty about that.

But whatever you do, keep motivating yourself and live a healthy life. You owe it to the most important person in your life: you!

Chapter Four

Getting NAKED with yourself

I have a reputation for being upfront and telling it like it really is. I have been told this could be seen as a detriment, but I am proud of my ability to tell it like it is no matter what. That has made me who I am, even if the person I have to confront is myself.

I knew that preparing myself for this diet was essential, and that I *must* keep to the diet if I wanted to succeed. I had set a goal of getting back down to eight percent body fat, which was where I was more than a decade ago when I was competing for the Mrs. Texas contests. But a lot had changed in my life and body since I won those competitions, and it was going to take real effort, teamwork and determination to get there.

My body had changed irrevocably after 30, and especially after 50, due to a natural change in hormone levels. A lot of diet books just don't approach this subject, or they gloss over it with a sentence or two. They certainly don't tell you that your dropping hormone levels as you age will affect your ability to work out and build muscle, your energy level and the way you store fat.

I am writing this book at the age of 54, so most of you are aware that my body has decreased its production of estrogen and begun menopause. This is when many women gain an extra ten to 15 pounds and find their waist thickens to a new dimension they have never experienced before, no matter how much they work out or cut back on calories. On top of this, many of us experience a health crisis related to aging, and this happened to me as well when I was in my early 50s. I was told I had to have a hysterectomy.

I recovered my energy and stamina well enough after my hysterectomy, but I found I couldn't seem to lose weight and my midsection was bloated for the first time in my life, no matter how hard I trained. After talking to my trainer and my doctor, I went on bioidentical hormones and have been able to retain my earlier physique and energy.

I learned a lot about hormones, diet and exercise from this experience, and I am going to share with you what has worked for me, with the understanding that it might not be right for everyone.

I have my hormone levels monitored consistently because hormones affect weight gain, as well as mood, which controls stress and sleep. It's all related. I am lucky enough to work with Heather Smith, my trainer's wife and co-owner of Sparta Fitness (and a former body builder), who is a licensed nurse practitioner specializing in women's wellness. She has guided me in my understanding of how hormone therapy works.

Progesterone affects your moods, sleep, headaches, PMS, and monthly cycles. Hormonal consistency avoids crashes. Testosterone builds muscle, which helps burn body fat and aids in cardio. Estrogen keeps the skin and breasts firm.

Heather explained to me that a whole generation of women has been placed on estrogen-dominant birth control, which has thrown their natural hormonal rhythms out of whack, and this may be part of the reason for the rise in obesity among younger and middle-aged women in this country.

Hormone replacement therapy has been part of the medical landscape for American women for decades now, and we have read the endless studies on whether it contributes to breast cancer and heart disease as well. But the hormone therapy most doctors prescribe is comprised of synthetic hormones created in a lab. I have opted to use bioidentical hormones, which are plant-based and all natural and have the same chemical structure as the hormones in your body. They were developed in the 1930s and are administered through pellets under the skin. They were overshadowed when synthetic hormones were created in the 1970s and could be taken as creams or pills, but they have a long, healthy, successful history of treatment with far fewer side effects than the more common chemical brands, which, of course, means they are not covered by insurance.

As a post-hysterectomy patient, you have to strengthen your core through exercise that includes targeted spot work on the abs and arms as well as cardio, a healthy high protein/low carb/no grain diet and ample hydration by drinking water.

In addition to regular hormone monitoring, women also have to watch their thyroid levels, as an underactive thyroid can lead to weight gain and decreased energy. Men can be affected by thyroid issues too, but they are much more common in women as they age.

So after you've been to your doctor and know your body's true condition, and you've faced the facts that there are still some biological factors you can't overcome by sheer will, you have to set realistic goals based on who you are and what you've been known to achieve. You have to stand naked in front a full-length mirror and see yourself as you really are, today.

In the appendix you'll find a one-page chart that asks you to examine the numbers of who you are at this moment. They include your weight, body measurements and body/fat ratio. The numbers may surprise you, but be honest.

As you stand in naked in front of that mirror, ask yourself, "Who am I? How did I get here? Who do I want to be?"

Hopefully, this book will help you answer those questions and get you to a place where you want to be.

Chapter Five

Getting Started

The basic tenet of this diet is to always be prepared. You should eat every three hours and you should never be hungry. Make sure you plan your meals.

A lot of dieters think they can skip breakfast, but breakfast really is one of the most important meals of the day. Since you will be working out quite hard on this program, it is imperative that you eat before you work out so you have the fuel and energy to reach your goals.

Do your shopping ahead of time, which means making sure you have whey protein on hand. Now this might sound like something you would dread eating, but it's come a long way since the days of Arnold Schwarzenegger and Lou Ferrigno. Today you can buy whey protein powder in an assortment of flavors that will astound you, from vanilla and chocolate to chocolate mint to peanut butter cup. My personal favorite is cookies and cream. When I combine it with cream of rice and a tablespoon of almond butter in the morning, it's like having dessert for breakfast! Buy a few different flavors so you aren't bored and have some variety. If you just cannot stand the whey, or it is causes you to have an upset stomach, an alternative is Raw Fit vegan protein powder by Garden of Life.

You also no longer need to go to a health food store or gym to buy protein powders. It's on sale everywhere, from CVS to Walmart as well as nutritional and health food stores, and can be easily ordered online.

You should also make sure you have Stevia or the brand Truvia on hand for sweetener, and that you have ordered your Udos supplement. I also like to have snacks such as rice cakes and crackers, as well as jars of almond or peanut butter. If you like popcorn, do not buy microwave popcorn, but buy whole kernels you will pop on the stove in a thin layer of oil.

In today's busy life, you can buy much of what you need to make this diet work, such as vacuum-packed chicken breasts or salmon pieces, in a simple run to your local Trader Joe's, Whole Foods or even online through Peapod or FreshDirect. Many of the foods you should stock up on are also available at Costco, Sam's Club and BJ's Wholesale Club too, so this diet doesn't have to cost you more than what you would normally spend.

You also need to be consistent on this plan to reach your goals. As I said, I like to exercise almost first thing in the morning because the boost I get from the endorphins puts me in a good mood all day. I have a colleague who works out at the end of the day, after work and dinner. She looks forward to this all day, as she thinks of it as her "me" time. Both of us plan our meals accordingly as well. I have my whey protein cream of rice breakfast before I work out. She has a yogurt/pineapple/banana/whey smoothie before she heads to the gym in the evening.

You also have to prepare your spirit for this change, and I have found the best way to do that is to look forward to it and make sure you have access to the relaxation tools and techniques that consistently work for you. As I have said, exercise (and its endorphin release) has been part of my wellbeing for years, but I also find comfort in reading. Many of my friends relax by listening to music, doing yoga, watching TV, playing video games, getting a massage and stretching. Just make sure you have ample time and access to these tools when you go on this diet.

You should take your measurements before you start the diet and fill them in on the chart in Appendix A so you can track your progress. Weigh yourself naked. Then begin measuring your percentage of body fat. You will see in the chart in Appendix A that there are two ways to do this. One uses a British measurement tool, the skinfold caliper, that squeezes your skin and fat together to measure its thickness. Among bodybuilders and fitness professionals, this is considered the more accurate way to measure a body/fat ratio, so I have included mine in the chart, and I will walk you through the measurement process (although you will need another person to do it with you, usually someone at your gym).

The second group of measurements are girth measurements, which are just taken in inches. This is where you will see the most consistent and striking results on this diet. Again, you might want to have someone else help you with taking the measurements because it is hard to get accurate measurements of areas like the space from shoulder to shoulder without another set of hands.

To calculate your percentage of body fat easily, you need to take your height and weight and enter it into a BMI calculator. BMI stands for body mass index. There is one online created by the federal government, so I am including that link here: http://www.nhlbi.nih.gov/health/educational/lose_wt/BMI/bmicalc.htm.

Not everyone needs to have a low percentage of body fat, but there are norms that vary due to gender, age and genetics. Of course, athletes will have a lower body fat percentage than the average person. The suggested healthy range for women between the ages of 30—50 is 15—23 percent. After 50, it is 16—25 percent. For men ages 30—50, it's 11—17 percent and 12—19 percent after 50. Women actually need more body fat than men.

The chart I've shared with you also tracks my percentage of muscle loss or gain, which is important to me because I was going for a leaner, stronger physique. You may not want to calculate these figures, but I am giving you the tools to do so, if you decide to. You measure muscle loss or gain by finding the weight of the lean mass by measuring the percentage of body fat and weight. To figure out the weight of the lean mass, when a person is weighed regularly, the amount lost (or gained) will represent the amount of muscle gained or lost.

My trainer has seen many men and women go on a variation of this diet and he has told me you should feel a change in your body and energy within 24—48 hours.

The following are additional items to get you off to the right start:

A very good blender—You've likely seen lots of ads for NutriBullet. This is an excellent blender, though a bit pricey. Look for one that has a lot of speed and sturdy blades.

A good water bottle and smoothie bottle—Blenderbottle.com makes a great bottle for blending varieties of liquids. The small metal BlenderBall® wire mixer makes sure there are no lumps or bumps in your liquid. You can also usually find plenty of water bottle models like this at your local grocery store.

Great sneakers for good back and leg support—This cannot be over-stated. You must have an excellent sneaker to take on the trauma from working out. Take your time and visit a few stores for fittings and recommendations. If you have a very high or no arch—two extremes—then you really need a sneaker that supports this.

Measuring spoons and measuring cups

Kitchen scale—This a great tool for weighing your food, especially the meats, to ensure you don't exceed the suggested weights. There are many selections on Amazon starting around $11. Type in "digital kitchen scale" in your search and you can spot one you love.

Fitness wear—While a good pair of sweat pants and a T-shirt may be fine, I suggest something that fits more snugly, yet comfortably, like Chaturanga leggings or Capris paired with a top that breathes.

NAKED IN 30 DAYS: PART TWO

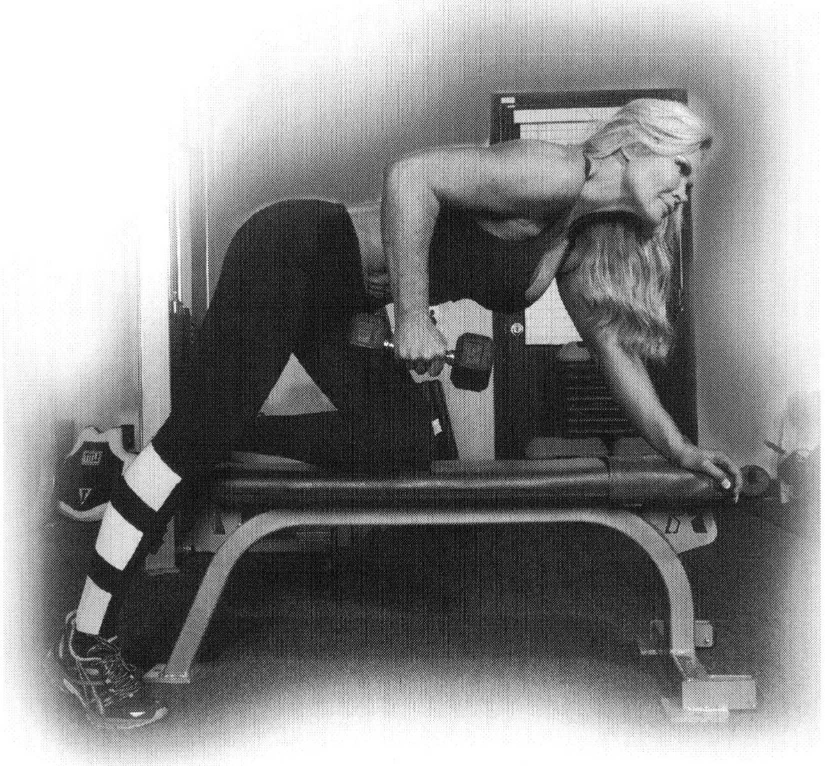

Day One

"No matter who you are, no matter what you did, no matter where you've come from, you can always change, become a better version of yourself."

—Madonna

The first day of exercise will consist of one hour of straight cardio followed by an abs exercise. I do one hour on a treadmill or an elliptical machine or I run for an hour. However, you might find one cardio exercise to be boring or monotonous, so feel free to break it up. There are plenty of cardio options available either at the gym or at home. You can hop on the treadmill or the elliptical machine, take a spin class, or if you enjoy running, get into a running regimen that includes walking briskly for 10—15 minutes and running for five minutes until you work your way up to a 30-minute or hour-long run. You can do an on-demand cardio video for 30 minutes, hop on the treadmill for a brisk 10-minute walk, jump on the elliptical for 10 minutes and back on the treadmill for another 10 minutes.

Have fun with it and challenge yourself. If you have been working out all along, then you know to make sure your workout breaks a sweat and that your heart rate should be in the fat-burning zone with interval bursts to get your heart rate up for brief periods of time. But, of course, pace yourself. However, if you haven't worked out in a while, make sure you start slow and build up your endurance each day.

Let's start off your first day of ab work with my preferred abdominal series:

Straight leg ab crunches
Lower ab crunches
Straight leg flutters
Abdominal crossover
V-ups
Resistance ball crunches
Ab rollers

Remember that you want to work up to three sets of 20 of each ab exercise. These are hard to do, so do as many as you can and be proud of what you have accomplished. Don't be frustrated if you can't do them all on the first day. Rome wasn't built in a day. Eventually you will get there.

NAKED Tip

Invest in a heart rate monitor like Fitbit, Polar, or Garmin that you can easily buy online. It is a useful tool to find your "sweet spot" target zone of heart beats per minute. The heart rate monitor is your pacer, telling you when to speed up or slow down to achieve the results you want to get with your workout.

NAKED Tip

Many people find it hard to stay motivated on their own, so try to recruit a friend to do this journey with you. Having someone to go to the gym with or go for a run with will help you stick to the plan for a longer time. You will count on each other to stay on track, and it will hold you accountable to the program. Once you make a plan with a friend, it's harder to back out at the last minute.

NAKED Tip

Variety is the spice of life, so mix up your cardio workouts and have fun with them. Boxing is a great cardio option that is also a form of resistance training and will help not only increase your endurance but strengthen and tone your full body. If you' re not sure what to do, join a boxing class, gym or download an on-demand boxing workout. There are lots of other great cardio options like swimming, hiking, or alternating running or walking up and down stairs.

Meal 1 (pre-workout)

Protein smoothies are a good meal before a workout because they are light, yet they give you the energy you need to work out.

1 scoop of protein powder shaken with 8 oz. of water.

NAKED Tip

Many of my NAKED followers and fans like to blend their protein powder with 1—2 cups of ice with almond milk instead of water. I'm old school. I don't mix it with ice, and I prefer the water. If you use the almond milk, try not to use the sweetened kind if you can avoid it. This may be tough starting out, so if you do use sweetened almond milk, try to mix half with water and/or wean yourself off over time.

NAKED Tip

I have a protein-rich shake with a cup of coffee with Stevia added in the morning. It gives me the energy I need to work out.

Meal 2 (post-workout)

¼ cup cream of rice cereal mixed in 1 cup of water

Boil the rice/water mixture in the microwave for about three minutes. If you use more water, the mixture is more watery like farina; less water and it's chunkier like a pudding. This is a personal preference, so you can discover which you prefer.

1 tsp of cinnamon sprinkled on top

Pinch of sea salt

NAKED Tip

The salt and cinnamon can be together or replace one another. Many people who follow me love to add a little sea salt and say it is delicious. You will find what you love.

Meal 3 (lunch salad with a protein)

1½ cup mixed greens, spinach, baby spinach, baby kale, or a mix of any two

6—8 oz. of lean meat

¼ cup of slivered almonds

1 tbsp. of dressing

NAKED Tip

You may find you need more dressing. If this is the case, add another tablespoon and try to wean yourself to less over time.

Meal 4 (snack)

1 rice cake with 1 tbsp. raw peanut butter or raw almond butter spread on top.

NAKED Tip

Rice cakes come in many flavors, including popcorn, Parmesan cheese, apple cinnamon and chocolate chip, to name a few. I love to spread my raw peanut butter or raw almond butter on a chocolate rice cake. It tastes like a Reese's peanut butter cup!

NAKED Tip

Alternate snacks include: ¼ cup of raw or roasted almonds (no salt!), ¼ cup of walnuts, ¼ cup of berries, or 1 apple.

Meal 5 (dinner)

6—8 oz. of salmon

Small side salad (e.g. 1 cup or less of spinach or kale) with chopped tomatoes and dressing

NAKED Tip

Squeeze some lemon on your salmon to give it some flavor, or even sprinkle some seasonings on while it bakes.

Meal 6 (optional, can replace another meal or be a snack)

¼ cup of nuts

½ cup of berries

or

1 cup of popcorn, air popped and no butter, okay to season with a tbsp. of herbs or spices

½ cup of berries

or

1 rice cake with 1 tbsp. of raw peanut butter or almond butter

¼ cup of berries

NAKED Tip

Remember, protein shakes are meals. If you are someone who works out at night instead of earlier in the day, you want to replace one of your meals with a protein shake before you work out to have the energy to burn.

Mind/spirit Tip: Take Baby Steps

One concept is essential to your mental, physical and spiritual approach to this journey. It underpins every chapter of this book, and it should guide your thought process as you get closer to the new, naked you: baby steps.

I'd love for everyone who reads this book to be running marathons and climbing mountains in 30 days, but that isn't how fitness works. That isn't how anything works. Forget the marathon for a second. The Chinese philosopher Lao Tzu is popularly credited with the saying, "A journey of a thousand miles begins with a single step." Before we learned how to run, we learned how to walk. Before that, we learned how to crawl. If you want to make progress toward a goal and you aren't sure where to start, don't focus on the end result. Focus on the first step. Start there.

As I'll explain in more depth later, unresolved grief can be a major impediment to your mental and spiritual health. If we never learn how to grieve, it can harm our physical well being. One revelation I had during the process of grieving my son's death was to focus on each moment. I prayed often every day. First, it was "God, just help me get through one hour of not crying." After I got through one hour, it became two hours. Then, an entire morning. People think they can lose someone and be better in a day, a week or a month, but it isn't going to happen. You're just a mess, all day long. Getting through every day was a matter of taking baby steps. I'd make it through half a day, then one day, then two, then one week. Then it became a month. To this day, I still go to church on the weekend and cry, bawling like a baby. Then I go back into the world, one hour at a time.

It's the same thing with diet and exercise. You can't lose 15 pounds overnight, or even in a week. The same baby steps you take when you begin to grieve are the same baby steps you take when you start a diet. Every elite marathoner started with a short run. Every elite weightlifter started with the lightest barbell in the gym.

Overcoming addictions is no different. Anyone who has been through recovery from drugs, alcohol or binge eating knows each day can be a struggle. Even one hour of sobriety can be a challenge. Maybe, hopefully, you've never been held captive by an addiction. The basic mechanism for changing any behavior pattern is always going to be the same: baby steps.

By repeating one successful hour 24 times a day, you can actually re-wire your brain to help achieve your goals. Shahram Heshmat, a professor at the University of Illinois-Springfield, explained how in an article for *Psychology Today*: "The core of an impulsive system is made of learned habits," Heshmat writes.

> "In the absence of self-control, habitual behavior is the default option. Especially when under the sway of overwhelming emotions, we react to surrounding cues without awareness of doing so. We fall back to our old habit whenever we face a stressful event. With each repetition, however, behavioral patterns become more automatic and part of an unconscious system."

You might not think you look good naked when you look in the mirror tomorrow. You might not feel better overnight. That's okay. Focus on the process, one baby step at a time, and the end result will come.

Day Two

"YOU are the only person standing in the way of
YOUR success!"
—Theresa Roemer

Today is your first full weight training workout along with abs. My trainer recommends starting with the upper body in a 45—60 minutes circuit. Changing estrogen levels make fat accumulate on the upper arms, especially toward the back of the arms, so this is an especially important series of exercises for women of a certain age.

Drink plenty of fluids throughout this workout, and make sure you drink after as well.

Before you begin, you need to warm up the upper body. One of my favorite stretching exercises is the **shoulder and arm warm up.**

Your upper body strength training workout will include a powerful circuit of exercises that focus on the shoulders, back and arms. Remember to start off with lighter weights, anywhere from 3—5 lbs. and work your way up to 8 lbs.

Circuit 1 (shoulder blast) standing or seated

Dumbbell (DB) front raise 12—15 reps
Side lateral-seated DB raises 12—15 reps
Seated DB presses 12—15 reps
DB upright rows 12—15 reps
Repeat circuit three to five times
Rest period 30—45 seconds

Circuit 2 (back and arms)

Tricep high lateral rope pull-downs 12—15 reps
Speed rows using band in squatting position 30—45 seconds
Tricep push-downs on cable machine 15—20 reps
Standing bicep DB curls 12—15 reps
Repeat circuit three to five times
Rest period 30—45 seconds

Circuit 3

One-arm DB row on flat bench 12—15 reps
Tricep kickbacks using DB 15—20 reps
Seated concentration DB curls 15—20 each arm
Repeat three to five times
Rest period 30—45 seconds

Circuit 4

Seated cable rows (machine) 12—15 reps
Standing tricep push-downs using tubing or bands 12—15 reps
Standing bicep curls 12—15 reps
Repeat three to five times
Rest period 30—45 seconds

At the end of your upper body workout, proceed to the abdominal circuit:

Straight legged ab crunches
Lower ab crunches
Straight leg flutters
Abdominal crossover
V-ups
Resistance ball crunches
Ab rollers

Remember that you want to work up to three sets of 20 of each ab exercise. Push yourself to do one or two more crunches than you did yesterday.

<u>NAKED Tip</u>

If you don't have dumbbells or are not comfortable using them at the gym or at home, invest in a good pair of resistance bands with handles. Resistance bands provide a smoother resistance exercise through the entire range of motion and are portable, so you can take them on the road if you are traveling. Be sure to start out with a lighter resistance and work your way up the heavy resistance bands. Bands can easily be purchased online.

<u>NAKED Tip</u>

If you can't make it to the gym and the workout specifies a weight training exercise to be done with a piece of equipment at the gym, swap it out with a similar exercise for that particular body part that you can easily do at home. For example, a tricep push-down on a cable machine can easily be done at home using a set of resistance bands tied to a stable door handle or staircase or do tricep dips. Most of the exercises I have described in the "Exercise" chapter of this book can be done at home so don't fret if you can't make it to the gym.

<u>NAKED Tip</u>

Start light. Lifting heavy weights with fewer repetitions ("reps") builds muscle size and mass, whereas lifting lighter weights with more reps tones muscles. Although you'll have to start off with lighter weights, don't get stuck in a routine where you keep lifting the same amount. *Gradually* increase the amount you lift.

Meal 1 (pre-workout)

Protein smoothie

1 scoop of protein powder shaken with 8 oz. of water.

<u>NAKED Tip</u>

Mix up your protein powders to find one or two you really love. Yesterday maybe you tried the vanilla, so today try the cookies and cream.

<u>NAKED Tip</u>

If you like your protein smoothies frothy, you can blend them in a blender with one or two cups of ice.

Meal 2 (post-workout)

2 whole eggs, 1 egg white (cage free), 1 oz. baby spinach, 1 tsp coconut oil to make omelet
⅛ tsp sea salt
¼ avocado

NAKED Tip

I am starving after my workout, so this is a very quick and filling meal. Sometimes I add a tablespoon of Parmesan cheese or diced tomatoes, and/or change the flavoring with garlic or cilantro.

Meal 3 (lunch salad with a protein)

1½ cup mixed greens, spinach, baby spinach, baby kale, or a mix of both
6—8 oz. of lean meat
¼ cup of slivered almonds
1 tbsp. of dressing

NAKED Tip

I love making turkey cutlets in advance for my lunch. I take the individual cutlets, dip them in a simple whipped egg batter, and shake to coat in a Ziplock bag of wheat bread crumbs and season to taste. Bake on a cookie sheet sprayed with coconut oil for 15—20 minutes. I make dozens of these and eat them throughout the week, on salads or even by themselves.

Meal 4 (snack)

1 rice cake with 1 tbsp. raw peanut butter or raw almond butter spread on top

NAKED Tip

Alternate snacks include: ¼ cup of raw or roasted almonds (no salt!), ¼ cup of walnuts, ¼ cup of berries or 1 apple.

Meal 5 (dinner)

6—8 oz. salmon
Small side salad (e.g. 1 cup or less of spinach or kale) with chopped tomatoes and dressing

NAKED Tip

I love salmon, but if you are not a fan, halibut, tilapia and cod are good options too.

Meal 6 (optional, can replace another meal or be a snack)

¼ cup of nuts

½ cup of berries

or

1 cup of popcorn, no butter, okay to season with a tbsp. herbs or spices

½ cup of berries

or

1 rice cake with 1 tbsp. of raw peanut butter or almond butter

½ cup of berries

NAKED Tip

Fruit is a tempting snack when so much sugar is removed from the diet. Try to limit your fruit and choose the most fibrous berries: blackberries, strawberries, blueberries.

Mind/Spirit Tip: Grieve

Of all the emotions, few have more power over the mind, body and spirit than grief. Grief can distract all our senses from the present moment. It can depress our spirits for days, weeks, months or years. If you're among the millions of Americans considered obese or overweight, there's an outstanding chance grief has contributed to the way your body looks today.

When my brother died at age 23, I had no way of knowing how to grieve. I was consumed by an empty feeling, thinking, "Now what?" My parents never told me "in case you ever encounter grief in your life, this is how to deal with it." Considering all the popular grief responses that are so much worse for your body, I can confidently say that fitness saved my life.

Many people are emotional eaters. I get it. Eating good food improves your mood. If your feelings are numb, food can become your best friend. It comforts you, like having someone put their arm around you. Sure, you might become overweight because of it, but food can be a consistent source of pleasure in dark moments. It doesn't talk back or say no. No police officer ever ordered you to put down a brownie.

Drugs and alcohol are closely related. They numb pain in the same way food comforts us. You can even drink at home, in your closet, where nobody is watching. In hindsight, I was lucky. I was never a big eater, and using alcohol and drugs to numb my grief never crossed my mind. The one thing I did know, and know well, was how to exercise.

Through experimentation, I found that when I did go to the gym, I felt better. When I wasn't unleashing my fury at God, I took out my anger in the aerobics room and the weight room. I was gainfully employed at a fitness center when my brother died. I became so close to the people who came to my classes, I would actually spend time crying with my class, talking about my brother. They all knew me, and I felt comfortable enough with them that I began pouring my emotions out. That was how I did it. That was how I grieved.

It wasn't working for my boss. One day he came to me and plainly said, "If you can't leave your emotions outside, I'm going to have to let you go." My boss pointed out something I would come to learn for myself in the years that followed: I wasn't the only one at the gym with grief. Everyone coming to my class had some emotional problem of their own to work out. They didn't need to add my stress to theirs.

"I need you to be the best actress in the world," my boss said. "You can cry all you want at home, but enter that door with a smile on your face. Be happy, be cheerful, lead a class, then pick your grief up on the way out the door."

Looking back, that was the best advice he could've given me. I learned something else in the process: the more I could share my story about my son, the more healing I experienced. My gym class wasn't the right setting, sure, but only by sharing our experiences with others can we truly grieve. Church groups, Bible study groups and grief groups offered me the comfort I needed without judgment—just like food, minus the calories.

If you're addicted to food, drugs or alcohol, and you don't know why, search your soul. Have you learned how to grieve? It's never too late to start sharing your story.

Day Three

"He that is good for making excuses is seldom good for anything else."
—Benjamin Franklin

We are halfway through the week, and ready for another day of cardio and abdominal exercise. Repeat the cardio workout you did on the first day, or switch it up. Aside from adding inclines, find other ways to make your cardio workout more challenging. Stand instead of resting your bottom on the seat when on your bike, run with high knees, or do the more intense butterfly stroke instead of the crawl. Remember that compared to the rest of your day, this workout is only a short time, so give it your all.

Finish your workout by completing the abs circuit:
Straight legged ab crunches
Lower ab crunches
Straight leg flutters
Abdominal crossover
V-ups
Resistance ball crunches
Ab rollers

Remember that you want to work up to three sets of 20 of each ab exercise. Push yourself to do one or two more crunches than you did yesterday.

NAKED Tip

Most forms of cardio are about the legs, so when possible, maximize your cardio time by focusing on working your arms as well. Swing them while running (don't hold on to the treadmill or elliptical handles), get creative with your arm strokes while in the pool, and don't forget to use them while in other cardio classes instead of resting them by your sides.

NAKED Tip

If running outside is not your cup of tea, and steep gym prices prevent you from hitting the pool or a spin class, you'll need an inexpensive and easy way to keep up with your cardio sessions. Jump ropes are a great tool to keep in your home gym. They're inexpensive (about $8), and for 30 minutes, a 130-pound woman can burn up to 330 calories. They are also portable so you can do your workout anywhere.

NAKED Tip

Don't forget to warm up before your workout. Doing a simple warm-up will increase mobility, decrease your chance of injury, and prepare your body's systems for the task at hand. Warm-ups are commonly overlooked, but skip them and you're bound to get hurt.

Meal 1 (pre-workout)

Protein smoothie

1 scoop of protein powder shaken with 8 oz. of water

NAKED Tip

Many people who blend their smoothies like to add a tablespoon of raw peanut butter to give it a peanut buttery taste. In this case you will want to use a blender to make sure it blends, particularly if water is your base.

Meal 2 (post-workout)

2 whole eggs, 1 egg white (cage free), 1 oz. baby spinach, 1 tsp coconut oil to make omelet

⅛ tsp sea salt

NAKED Tip

Eggs have earned a bad reputation due to their high cholesterol content, which was at one time associated with heart disease. It is only fairly recently that medical professionals have learned that cholesterol is not the main cause of this, but rather the saturated fats that have a much more adverse effect on blood cholesterol. Saturated fats live in fatty meats and full-fat dairy products. The saturated fats are what trigger the body to produce cholesterol.

Meal 3 (lunch salad with a protein)

1 can of white tuna in water

1 cup mix of chopped broccoli, cauliflower, red onion and celery

Mix ¼ cup of olive oil with 3 tablespoons lemon juice, 2 tablespoons soy sauce, 1 tsp mustard.

NAKED Tip

The dressing above is a wonderful and healthy alternative to mayonnaise. I also add salt and pepper to taste.

Meal 4 (snack)

2 celery stalks with raw peanut butter or raw almond butter

NAKED Tip

Celery is a great snack, not only because it gives you that crunch you crave, but has so many health benefits, including the fact it's a good antioxidant to protect our bodies from oxidative damage, which is an imbalance between the production of free radicals and the body's ability to detoxify their harmful effects. It is also a great anti-inflammatory food and particularly good for your intestinal track.

Meal 5 (dinner)

6—8 oz. lean turkey

1 cup of boiled broccoli, Brussels sprouts or cauliflower

NAKED Tip

Broccoli, Brussels sprouts and cauliflower are packed with nutrients and known to help boost the immune system

Meal 6 (optional, can replace another meal or be a snack)

¼ cup of nuts
½ cup of berries
or
1 cup of popcorn, no butter, okay to season with a tbsp. herbs or spices
½ cup of berries
or
1 rice cake with 1 tbsp. of raw peanut butter or almond butter
¼ cup of berries

NAKED Tip

Cranberries and strawberries are rich in quercetin, which has a strong anti-inflammatory effect on the body.

Mind/Spirit Tip: Meditate

I'm not a guru, or a yogi, or an expert in meditation in any traditional sense. In fact, my experience with meditation has taught me that you don't need a great deal of expertise to reap its benefits. Simplicity is at the heart of what makes meditation great.

What might be the most difficult aspect of meditating for some of you is also the most important: finding a quiet area in which you can be alone. For me, that might be a corner of a room, a pew in church, a shady tree trunk, or a chair by a window. These are all places you can find everywhere, no matter where work or life takes you. Close your eyes. Breathe. Empty your mind of your thoughts, your anxiety and whatever might be causing you stress in that moment.

What more can be said about meditation that hasn't already been put to paper? Some of the earliest writings on the topic have been traced to 1500 B.C. in India. If you want more information, it's out there. The pace of life in ancient India was certainly slower than wherever you happen to be living right now. If anything, meditation is even more essential today as a respite from our daily lives. Eighteen million Americans would agree, according to the most recent statistics from the Department of Health and Human Services.

One of the 18 million is a neuroscientist at Massachusetts General Hospital and Harvard Medical School named Sara Lazar. As she explained to *The Washington Post* in 2015, she was stretching in a yoga class, preparing to run the Boston Marathon, when the teacher introduced her to meditation. She felt better for it, so she decided to study the effects of meditation on the human brain. Here's what Lazar found:

> 1. Long-term meditators had more gray matter in their auditory and sensory cortex than people in a control group. They also had more gray matter in their frontal cortex, which is associated with working memory and executive decision-making.
> 2. In a study comparing prefrontal cortexes, 50-year-old meditators had the same amount of gray matter as 25-year-olds.
> 3. In a study comparing two groups, one that consisted of novices who meditated for eight weeks and another group of non-meditators, the meditators had enlarged brains.
> 4. The group of meditators in the latter experiment had smaller amygdalas, an area of the brain that regulates stress, compared to their non-meditating counterparts.

Lazar made no claims about a connection between meditation and happiness, but Matthieu Ricard does. Dubbed by the media as the "world's happiest man," Ricard is a practicing Tibetan Buddhist monk. When meditating, his brain produced more gamma rays than ever recorded in neuroscience literature. Imagine the eight-week meditators with enlarged brains, then multiply those effects out over 50 years. That's Ricard. He says he meditates for entire days without getting bored.

You probably don't have time to set aside entire days for meditation. That's okay. The beauty of meditating is that it can be done anytime, anyplace and by anyone. You don't have to believe in God to benefit from the quiet solitude of sitting in a church pew. You don't even have to like being in nature to find calm sitting under a tree. What you do with that quiet, meditative time is up to you. Some like to pray. Some like to focus on breathing. Some like to let their thoughts flow and see where it takes them. For me, running outdoors can serve the same purpose as sitting quietly. It relaxes me and focuses my thoughts.

The purpose, for me, is to slow the pace of life for a portion of your day. It'll make you a happier person. Your heart rate will thank you in the moment, and your enlarged brain will return the favor for years to come.

66

Day Four

"I attribute my success to this—I never gave or took any excuse."
—Florence Nightingale

Today we are going to focus on working the lower body, which will include leg and buttock exercises. Before we begin, it's a good idea to do some stretching to get your muscles warmed up and ready to go. I like to start with the hamstring glute stretch and the lower back stretch. Keep in mind that the recommended set amounts are what you want to work up to. Start slow and do what you can. What you do today is better than doing nothing at all.

Drink plenty of water, and don't forget to complete your workout with the abdominal circuit.

Lower body circuit (45—60 minutes)
Five-minute warm up
Leg extensions 15—20 reps, four sets

Circuit 1
Smith machine squats 15—20 reps
Walking lunges 50—75 yards
Seated or kneeling leg curls machine 15—20 reps
Repeat 3—4 sets
Rest period 30—45 seconds

Circuit 2

Seated leg press (machine) 15—20 reps
Standing body weight squats 30—40 reps
Anterior reach lunge 12—15 each leg
Repeat four to five times
Rest period 30—45 seconds

Circuit 3

Jump squats 30 seconds
Alternating jumping lunges 30 seconds
Repeat three to four times
Rest period 30—45 seconds

Circuit 4

Lying glute bridge off stability ball, legs straight, 15—20 reps
Lying glute bridge with knees bent, feet flat on ball, pushing hips up as high as you can, 15—20 reps
Lying leg curls on stability ball 15—20 reps
Repeat three to four times
Rest period 30—45 seconds

NAKED Tip

For a proper squat technique use an athletic stance for the squat so your knees are slightly bent, your feet are firmly planted on the ground, and your toes pointed outward slightly, which helps with stabilization. The wider you put your feet, the more it works your glutes and hamstrings (back of the leg), and the easier it will be to stabilize. The closer in you put your feet, the more your quadriceps will be emphasized (the front of the leg).

NAKED Tip

Even though lunges are one of the best ways to work your lower body, some people tend to avoid them because they can put too much strain on the knees. If you feel pain, take smaller steps. Slowly increase your lunge distance as your pain decreases. Some people also find doing a reverse lunge instead of a forward lunge also helps reduce knee strain.

NAKED Tip

It's necessary to wear proper footwear with good support when conducting lower-body strength-training exercises. When you work out, especially during leg exercises you have to be driving through the heels. Do not wear running shoes. The sole does not support that and will cause you to lose stability. Lifting shoes or cross-training shoes can help you to feel sturdier during squats and deadlifts.

Meal 1 (pre-workout)

Protein smoothie

1 scoop of protein powder shaken with 8 oz. of water.

NAKED Tip

A fan once wrote to me that he likes to sprinkle instant coffee powder on top of his smoothies to give his workout a kick. Hey, if it works for you, go for it!

Meal 2 (post-workout)

Awesome omelet

1 large egg

4 egg whites, cage-free

½ tsp. sea salt

1 tablespoon freshly chopped cilantro

¼ cup chopped onion

¼ cup black beans

¼ cup tomatoes

NAKED Tip

I like to make this omelet to change things up. You can also simply scramble the eggs with the cilantro, sea salt, onions and beans, or just scramble the eggs and mix the other ingredients in.

Meal 3 (lunch salad with a protein)

1 can of white tuna in water

1 cup mix of chopped broccoli, cauliflower, red onion and celery

Mix ¼ cup of olive oil with 3 tablespoons lemon juice, 2 tablespoons soy sauce, 1 tsp mustard.

NAKED Tip

Why do health care professionals like to promote tuna? Because tuna is high in Omega-3 fatty acids, which help to reduce cholesterol in the arteries and blood vessels, which in turn helps reduce coronary heart disease.

Meal 4 (snack)

2 celery stalks with raw peanut butter or raw almond butter

NAKED Tip

You will notice I like to make foods with raw peanut butter. The reason is that this is a good fat, considered a monounsaturated fat, which helps decrease cardiovascular disease risk.

Meal 5 (dinner)

6—8 oz. flank steak, cooked to taste
1½ cups baby kale
1 cup chopped tomatoes
Salt and pepper to taste

NAKED Tip

Flank steak can be prepared on a grill or simply seared in a pan on the stove. You can have your baby kale and tomatoes by themselves or top this salad with the flank steak for a tasty flank steak salad.

Meal 6 (optional, can replace another meal or be a snack)

¼ cup of nuts
½ cup of berries
or
1 cup of popcorn, no butter, okay to season with a tablespoon of herbs or spices
½ cup of berries
or
1 rice cake with 1 tablespoon of raw peanut butter or almond butter
¼ cup of berries

NAKED Tip

Prunes are a sweet snack you might enjoy as a dessert or snack earlier in the day, as they are a good source of energy and high in fiber. They also do not contribute to a rise in blood sugar.

Mind/Spirit Tip: Sleep

As a single mom running my own business, I made a habit of getting two to four hours of sleep a night for years. Deep down I knew that wasn't healthy, but since I had to do it, I pushed through. In some ways it wasn't hard. I'm not someone who likes to turn my mind off. The ideas might be racing at 1:00 in the morning, well past my bedtime, but why sleep when I can get work done?

In the long term, that attitude isn't healthy. These days I aim to get a good seven to eight hours a night. Learning how to sleep that much was a process for me. I had to train my brain to relax long enough that it could turn off at night. For some, good sleep habits come naturally. For me, it was a skill I had to master.

One epiphany in particular set me on the path to a better night's sleep, the light bulb in my head that got me to turn off the light bulb on my nightstand: just because a problem is on your mind when you're lying in bed wide awake, doesn't mean you can solve it right then and there. One night, I was lying awake from midnight until 4:00 a.m. All the cares in the world were running through my head. The old Theresa would have said, "Okay, let's get up and tackle the world right now!" Instead, I decided to stay in bed. I tried to banish the bothersome thoughts. It wasn't pretty. I forced myself to lie in bed for an hour and a half, talking to myself and turning on my sides. I couldn't fall asleep until 5:30. Two hours later I was awake. That's not ideal, of course, but it was a night I could chalk up to the learning process.

So, how much sleep should you get? The general answer is seven to eight hours, but the ideal amount of sleep will differ for each of you. Circadian rhythms—our "body clock" that affects sleep, jetlag, body temperature and hormone release—have a genetic component. Since we all have different genes, no specific number works for everyone. However, a lot of sleep research offers more concrete lessons.

If you have chronic insomnia, the National Sleep Foundation says exercise is one of the best things you can do. If nothing else, follow the 30-day exercise plan in this book and your sleep might improve. Where exercise habits go, dietary habits tend to follow, and that's true for sleep as well. Alcohol, cigarettes and caffeine can all disrupt a good night's sleep. Eating big or spicy meals can cause discomfort from indigestion, making it harder to sleep. The National Sleep Foundation recommends avoiding large meals for two to three hours before bedtime, with a light snack 45 minutes before bedtime if you're still hungry.

Another tip: turn off your electronic devices long before you tuck in for the night. Research shows even the small glow of a smartphone essentially tricks your brain into thinking it's daytime, promoting wakefulness. If you're having trouble sleeping, playing a game or reading something on your phone is one of the worst things you can do.

In those moments, I turn my attention to light thoughts. Grandchildren. Happy times. Anything that slows down my heart rate. I keep the light turned off and push through until my body and brain have stopped fidgeting. When it's time for bed, all the world's problems can wait until tomorrow.

Day Five

“Success is not final, failure is not fatal: it is the courage to continue that counts.”
—Winston S. Churchill

Your body may be tired and a little sore, but I am sure you can already feel the difference in your energy level. It’s amazing how working out invigorates you even as it exhausts you.

Today is another day of cardio and ab exercises. Don’t forget to stretch your muscles before your workout. If you don’t, you will feel it five minutes into your workout.

NAKED Tip

Know your target heart rate (THR). This is a must, because if you’re under your target heart rate, you’re not doing much to get yourself ripped. The actual equation is subtract your age from 220, but use that heart rate monitor I suggested in Day One.

NAKED Tip

Running is one of the best calorie-burning forms of cardio training. To try something different, and to challenge your body in a new way, try adding hills to your workout routine. Hill running is a great way to get your heart working as well as to challenge the lower-body muscles. Find a hill that takes about 15—20 seconds to run up and repeat five or six times during your workout session.

NAKED Tip

If spinning is your preferred form of cardio, today try transitioning between a seated and standing position to maximize results. Adding one to two-minute standing intervals to your spinning routine will target the muscles from a slightly different angle as you move throughout the workout and ensure you get the full benefits the exercise has to offer.

Meal 1 (pre-workout)

Protein smoothie

1 scoop of protein powder shaken with 8 oz. of water.

NAKED Tip

Sometimes the full protein smoothie may seem like too much before a tough workout. If you feel too full, simply only have half the protein smoothie and save the other half as an additional treat for your post-workout meal or breakfast.

Meal 2 (post-workout)

2 eggs, 1 egg white (cage free) for scrambled eggs or omelet with:

¼ cup chopped red onion

½ chopped green pepper

⅓ cup spinach

NAKED Tip

Pairing spinach with eggs is smart. Spinach is high in calcium for bone health, iron for preventing anemia, magnesium for proper muscle function, and vitamin A for healthy vision. Eggs are high in vitamin B-12, which helps in preventing nerve damage, and vitamin D, which helps your body absorb calcium.

Meal 3 (lunch salad with a protein)

6—8 oz. grilled skinless chicken breast

1½ cup mixed greens, spinach, baby spinach, baby kale, or a mix of both

¼ cup of slivered almonds

1 tbsp. of dressing

NAKED Tip

Chicken has many wonderful benefits and satisfies your appetite for long periods of time. It's high in protein and helps build muscle. The calcium in chicken helps keep bones healthy. It has lots of trace minerals to boost your immune system. It's rich in selenium, which cuts the risk of developing arthritis; and it is rich in vitamin B5, which has a calming effect on the nerves—nothing like some good chicken to help you chill out!

Meal 4 (snack)

1—2 cups of kale to make crispy kale chips
Spread raw kale leaves on a cookie sheet sprayed with olive oil
Drizzle 1 tablespoon of olive oil over the kale leaves and top with pinch of sea salt
Cook at 375 degrees until crispy

NAKED Tip

Kale is a clever green and packed with health benefits. It is a member of the cabbage family and one of the most nutrient-dense foods around. It is packed with antioxidants to counteract oxidative damage, known to be a leading driver in aging and diseases including cancer. It helps lower blood pressure, contributes to heart health, and is an anti-inflammatory, anti-viral, and natural anti-depressant.

Meal 5 (dinner)

6—8 oz. grilled skinless chicken breasts, sliced into strips
1—2 cups mixed greens
¼ red onion, sliced for long, thin slices
½ cup black beans
1 tablespoon dressing

NAKED Tip

Little tweaks to your simple menu of lean meats and greens help keep your diet a little more interesting. Try slicing your chicken into long slices and placing them atop a bed of greens with long, thin slices of red onion and then sprinkle with black beans. Drizzle your favorite dressing on top.

Meal 6 (optional, can replace another meal or be a snack)

¼ cup of nuts
½ cup of berries
or
1 cup of popcorn, no butter, okay to season with a tbsp. herbs or spices
½ cup of berries
or
1 rice cake with 1 tbsp. of raw peanut butter or almond butter
¼ cup of berries

<u>NAKED Tip</u>

Popcorn is a great source of antioxidants and fiber. It's when you add butters and caramels that it becomes unhealthy. Try it raw or sprinkle with garlic, Parmesan or a little sea salt.

Mind/Spirit Tip: Ask for Help

One of the byproducts of looking good naked is a healthy ego, so maybe the concept of asking for help seems out of place in this book. Just bear with me. Sometimes a little help is exactly the thing your body, mind and spirit needs. It's an important skill that just might save your life.

As a little girl, the one lifeline I always had was with my mother. She seemed to have a solution to every problem in the world. Even as an adult, my relationship with my mom didn't change. Whenever I encountered a situation I couldn't quite handle—a medical issue, a question about raising children, or any of life's little lessons—I would automatically pick up the phone and call her. Mom was my go-to person, a walking encyclopedia. With her, I never thought of it as asking for help. She's the world's problem solver.

If only we were always so comfortable asking for help when we needed it. As a trainer, I've worked with people who were at the top of their profession: big-time engineers, architects and others who seem to have the world by the tail. For an amazingly accomplished person, sometimes admitting you need help takes a lot of guts. Maybe you built a skyscraper but don't have the first idea of how to lose weight. That's okay! We can't all know how to do everything. I've worked with Ph.D.'s who were 40 pounds overweight. In the 30-plus years I've been a certified trainer, I've asked many people who were badly out of shape why they didn't seek help sooner. The excuse I heard most often was, "You don't even know how hard it was to ask for help. I feel like a failure."

For some of you, the act of asking for professional help might be the number-one thing that stands in the way of looking and feeling good naked. That isn't limited to people who are obese, overweight or out of shape. Alcoholics, drug addicts and people struggling with certain mental health issues (like depression) are powerless on their own against forces that can ruin a person's life. Those are all examples of issues that carry dire consequences if left untreated. But diseases related to obesity can kill you just the same. By committing to the program contained in these pages, you've already done the hardest thing for many people: you've admitted you need help and done something about it.

At some point, all of us will need help doing things that came easier when we were younger—including but not limited to losing weight. We shouldn't feel embarrassed about that. That's normal. According to Dr. Ellen Hendriksen, a clinical psychologist at Stanford University, many of us fear asking for help because we don't want to burden others. But people love to help! "The most primitive part of the brain, the same reward pathway activated by food and sex, lights up in response to altruistic giving," Hendriksen wrote in *Scientific American*. "Graciously allow your helper to give you a gift of help; she or he will likely be delighted for the chance."

Asking for help is a skill you can practice every day. Start small. Burdened by stress at work? Ask a colleague you trust. Burdened by housework? Ask your husband, your children or even a neighbor. A little help might go a long way. Your body, mind and spirit will reap the benefits. That's why asking for help shouldn't be a blow to your ego. It can actually be a major boost!

Day Six

"Desire is the key to motivation, but it's determination and commitment to an unrelenting pursuit of your goal—a commitment to excellence—that will enable you to attain the success you seek."
—Mario Andretti

We return to the upper body series of exercises today, which will target the chest, shoulders and back. Developing strength and endurance in these areas will enhance your overall appearance as well as your health. You will be surprised by not only how much better you look, but by how much better you feel. If you do these workouts the right way, your posture will improve, and those back pains you had will disappear!

It is important to get your heart going, so start by warming up. You want to ensure your whole body is ready to work out. Warming up is essential in ensuring that you are able to move as you should without a high risk of injuries.

Some of the warm-up exercises you can do to get yourself going include marching on the spot, walking briskly, jumping rope, push-ups and so on. The key is to get your body gradually accustomed to intense movements.

Drink plenty of water and don't forget to complete your workout with the abdominal circuit.

Circuit 1 (back)
Lat pull-downs 3 sets of 15 reps
Seated rows 3 sets of 15 reps
Assisted pull-ups 3 sets of 15 reps
Repeat three to five times
Rest period 30—45 seconds

Circuit 2 (chest)

Standard push-ups 20 reps
Dumbbell presses, three sets of 15
Reverse push-ups on the rubber ball to failure
Repeat three to five times
Rest period 30—45 seconds

Circuit 3 (shoulders)

Dumbbell (DB) Front Raise 12—15 reps
Side Lateral Seated DB Raises 12—15 reps
Seated DB Presses 12—15 reps
DB Upright Rows 12—15 reps
Repeat circuit three to five times.
Rest period 30—45 seconds

NAKED Tip

Take time to cool down so your body can adjust to its normal pace again. Stretching exercises come in handy during this time because they help remove the stiffness from your body and keep injuries at bay.

NAKED Tip

If you're a beginner and you can't perform a standard push-up with good form, start with knee push-ups. Work your way up until you complete 20—25 repetitions with good form. This means keeping your hips in line with your body and not letting the hips sag toward the floor or pushing your butt up toward the ceiling. Once you can do at least 20 good knee push-ups, move to standard push-ups. Start with as many repetitions as you can with good form, then move to bent knee push-ups to do a total of about 20 push-ups. Gradually increase the number of standard push-ups until you can complete an entire set.

NAKED Tip

Enlist a training partner when doing dumbbell presses so he or she can give you a few forced reps at the end of each set. That means you do the first number of reps on your own, to failure, and then have your partner force you to do three to five more. Your partner can either grab your wrists or under your elbows. Having them spot grab your wrists can avoid the dumbbell from crashing down on you plus you get the benefits of doing extra reps.

Meal 1 (pre-workout)

Protein smoothie

1 scoop of protein powder shaken with 8 oz. of water.

NAKED Tip:

You will likely want to weigh yourself tomorrow, which is day seven, and then celebrate with a cheat day when you see how far you've come. Today's program mirrors day one because it is very minimal and we don't want to load up before a weigh in.

Meal 2 (post-workout)

¼ cup cream of rice cereal mixed in 1 cup of water

Boil the rice/water mixture in the microwave for about three minutes. If you use more water, the mixture is more watery like farina, less water and it's chunkier like a pudding.

1 tsp of cinnamon sprinkled on top

Pinch of sea salt

Meal 3 (lunch salad with a protein)

1½ cup mixed greens, spinach, baby spinach, baby kale or a mix of both

6—8 oz. of lean meat

¼ cup of slivered almonds

1 tbsp. of dressing

NAKED Tip

A friend loves this vinaigrette dressing. 1 tbsp. red wine vinegar, ⅓ tsp. sea salt, 1 tbsp mustard, 3 tbsp olive oil, 1 tsp. pepper.

Meal 4 (snack)

1 rice cake with 1 tbsp. raw peanut butter or raw almond butter spread on top.

NAKED Tip

Rice cakes are low in fat, calories and sugar. While they don't give you huge amounts of vitamins or minerals, they are a quick and easy snack.

NAKED Tip

Alternate snacks include: ¼ cup of raw or roasted almonds (no salt!), ¼ cup of walnuts, ¼ cup of berries, or 1 apple.

Meal 5 (dinner)

6—8 oz. of salmon

Small side salad (e.g. 1 cup or less of spinach or kale) with chopped tomatoes and dressing

NAKED Tip

Salmon is well known to have many benefits and recent studies have found it contains bioactive peptides that may support joint cartilage, control inflammation in the digestive tract and help counter insulin resistance, which is when the normal amount of insulin secreted into the bloodstream is not sufficient to move glucose to the cells to be used for fuel.

Meal 6 (optional, can replace another meal or be a snack)

¼ cup of nuts

½ cup of berries

or

1 cup of popcorn, air popped and no butter, okay to season with a tbsp. herbs or spices

½ cup of berries

or

1 rice cake with 1 tbsp. of raw peanut butter or almond butter

¼ cup of berries

NAKED Tip

Studies have shown that when you eat late at night, the body is more likely to store calories and fat, rather than burning it for energy.

Mind/Spirit Tip: Connect with Others

Your mind and spirit cannot flourish on their own. Making deep, lasting connections with other human beings is just as essential to your health as any diet or exercise plan. Twenty percent of Americans identified loneliness as a source of suffering in one survey, and when we suffer we're less likely to take care of ourselves. We're hard-wired to be connected and when we're disconnected, it's painful. Neuroscience tells us the emotional reaction to rejection emanates from the same area of our brain that responds to physical pain. That's why a broken heart can hurt just as much as a broken leg.

The number of Americans living alone is only rising, so the need to connect is especially important now. If you can't come home to anyone in your support system, it's critical you make the effort to assemble that network. Without a group of people who have your back, a lot of the wisdom contained in this book will be useless. You'll have no one to grieve with, no one you can ask for help, and no one to tell you when you're not dressed for success.

When I was a fitness instructor, sharing the pain over losing my brother in class wasn't the right time or place to grieve. But guess what? It helped immensely. Even those of you who are living alone can do what I (eventually) did in those dark times: join a Bible study or a grief-support group; the website griefshare.org is a fantastic resource. Don't know anyone who shares your common interests? Check out the website Meetup.com. It exists just for people just like you. You can even start a "meetup group" for people who want to read this book and go through the 30-day program together. Your chances of sticking to the program will only increase, I promise.

It's important to include others in becoming a new you. Everyone needs a group of trusted friends who can serve as accountability partners. They're the ones who can tell you when they think you're being abused by someone else, or when you need to let go of that ax to grind. Your body is limited by its physical dimensions, but no mind or spirit ever existed in a vacuum. We're all in this together.

And yet, research shows our instinct is to ignore strangers, even though we're much happier when we strike up a conversation with them. We aren't even any less productive. You can make all the excuses you want to refrain from putting yourself out there in the world—I'll have more on excuses in a later chapter—but it literally makes no sense to give in. You're a much healthier person in the presence of others who you can relate to. Having friends means you're less likely to turn to food for comfort in times of stress, as studies show a high correlation between obesity and loneliness. Being connected to other people only makes it easier to lose weight and, ultimately, feel better naked.

When my marriage ended, I felt very alone in the world. If I'd had a better support system at the time, I probably would have had the self-esteem to put my foot down sooner, knowing I deserved better than the abuse my first husband was inflicting. It's natural to fear the pain that comes with feeling rejected by another person, but don't let that be your excuse. Being isolated, or being stuck in a codependent relationship with another person, will only hurt you more in the long run.

Day Seven—Cheat Day!

"Most folks are as happy as they make up their minds to be."
—Abraham Lincoln

Congratulations! You've made it to your rest day and the end of the first week on the program.

If you're like me, you can't sit still on a rest day. Although rest is needed to give some time for the body to recuperate, it is still important to remain active on those days. The body, just like the mind, needs stimulation every day so go for a walk, take the stairs or do static stretch exercises.

You are going to repeat the program and the daily menus for the next three weeks with some variation. There are going to be days when you don't feel like working out, and when you feel you would really like a piece of bread in a restaurant or a slice of cake, but know that if you give in, it will take that much longer to reach your goal. Once you have gone through a week, your body has already acclimated to the exercise and dietary changes.

But even if you do give in, or skip a day of exercise, get back on the diet right away. You need to forgive yourself and try again.

NAKED Tip

The biggest problem most people have with rest days is that they treat them as cheat days! Because they're not training, they're not thinking about being fit, and it's much easier to slack off and lose momentum. For that reason, one of the best things you can do on an off day is to work on your flexibility and mobility. After all, what good is strength if we can't move our body properly to utilize it! Dynamic stretching and mobility work, like yoga and Pilates, aids in muscle recovery, helps prepare our body for the rigors of strength training and keeps us injury-free!

NAKED Tip

Spend your rest days working on your happiness and having fun at the same time. Take in a movie with your family, friends or loved ones, but park in the farthest spot in the parking lot. Go for a bike ride with your kids or gather your neighbors for an impromptu softball game. Spending time with those you love will keep you happy and motivated.

NAKED Tip

A weekly massage would be great for your body but not so great for your wallet. Instead, invest in a foam roller for some do-it-yourself muscle relief. This self-massaging technique loosens stiff muscles and helps keep muscles loose. Foam rolling, along with stretching and cross-training, can help prevent repetitive stress injuries that could disrupt training. Aim to roll at least once or twice a week. Your body will thank you.

Mind/Spirit Tip: Express Gratitude

One of the greatest lessons my parents taught me as a little girl was the importance of giving thanks. It wasn't so much a lesson as a habit my siblings and I accepted as a part of life. Right after Christmas every year, we all wrote thank-you letters to the people who gave us a gift: aunts, uncles, grandparents—everyone.

I can honestly say I've taken this practice even more seriously as I've gotten older. It makes sense if you think about it: as a child, your world is much smaller, with relatively few people helping you navigate life. Now, as an adult, you've forged many relationships over the years. Wherever you might be in life, there are plenty of folks who have helped you get there. You've collected more people, things and experiences to be thankful for. I can't begin to compare the number of "thank you" letters (including emails) I send today to the number I sent when I was a child.

Unfortunately, I meet people who either never made expressing gratitude a habit or lost that good habit along the way. Now, when I give someone a gift, I have to brace for the possibility that they might not acknowledge receiving it at all. That's just as unhelpful as it is disrespectful. Was the gift ever delivered? If you're not sure, you might have to send an email or text message just to make sure the delivery service did its job. Any acknowledgement that you received a gift is better than nothing.

Psychologist Susan Krauss Whitbourne, writing on the website PsychologyToday.com, says thank-you notes should be "short, sweet, and easy to write." Don't feel like you have to write something long and worthy of a Nobel Prize in Literature. That's not the point of expressing gratitude. The less pressure you put on yourself, the less likely you are to put it off.

Expressing gratitude is so beneficial in so many hidden ways, it's a practice that shouldn't wait until you receive a gift. We can all practice expressing gratitude daily. A team of psychologists once ran an experiment in which people were asked to keep a weekly journal of things for which they were grateful. The subjects reported higher levels of alertness, enthusiasm, determination, optimism and energy, along with less depression and stress. They were more likely to help others, *exercise* and make progress toward personal goals. The research suggested that "anyone can increase their sense of wellbeing and create positive social effects just from counting their blessings."

These effects are blind to your religion, even though it's worth noting that every major religion has something to say about being kind to others. Gratitude feeds your mind, body and spirit regardless of your beliefs.

I don't keep a physical gratitude diary. But if you're someone who expresses thanks daily, your life essentially becomes a living gratitude diary. There's never a bad time to pick up the phone and say "thank you." Not sure where to start? Author and entrepreneur Tim Ferriss recommends asking one question every morning when you wake up—what am I truly grateful for in my life?—and aim for five answers.

Receiving thanks and praise from someone can really lift your spirits. It's reassuring to know that giving thanks and praise can do the same!

Day Eight

"What you do today can improve all your tomorrows."
—Ralph Marston

Today is the start of your second week on my program. It's a cardio day, so start the week off right and push yourself to run faster, swim harder or increase your resistance in a spin class. The nice thing about cardio exercise is that you can choose any activity that raises your heart rate. You don't have to do the same workout every session, or every week. If you've been doing the same workouts, you'll likely get bored. Changing up your cardio is easy, so do it often and you'll discover more activities you enjoy.

Being active can make our lives better. Moving around increases blood flow to our muscles, strengthens the heart and lungs and teaches the heart to work more efficiently. Not only that, when you exercise you start to feel better about yourself, and that confidence can carry you through to that next workout when you feel tired or too sore to keep going.

Round out your cardio workout with the abdominal series:
Straight leg ab crunches
Lower ab crunches
Straight leg flutters
Abdominal crossover
V-ups
Resistance ball crunches
Ab rollers

Remember that you want to work up to three sets of 20 of each ab exercise. Push yourself to increase your reps and really feel the burn.

NAKED Tip

Try to learn to appreciate your body. Just taking a few moments during your workouts to imagine what it would be like if you couldn't do what you wanted can help remind you how amazing your body is—no matter how it looks.

NAKED Tip

If you're lacking motivation to finish your workout, use a visual reminder. Picture yourself finishing your workout. Not only that, imagine yourself gliding through it effortlessly, feeling satisfied, proud of yourself, confident and ready to face the rest of the day. Just the thought of your body operating like a well-oiled machine can change your posture and, perhaps, even your perception of how your body feels.

Meal 1 (pre-workout)

Protein smoothie

1 scoop of protein powder shaken with 8 oz. of water.

NAKED Tip:

You can sweeten your protein shake with Stevia or Truvia, and some fans have written they take a tablespoon of honey and mix it in, particularly if they are using a blender with ice to make a frothier smoothie.

Meal 2 (post-workout)

¼ cup cream of rice cereal mixed in 1 cup of water

Boil the rice/water mixture in the microwave for about 3 minutes.

NAKED Tip

Another good alternate to the cream of rice cereal is oatmeal. Oatmeal is a great source of fiber and contains potassium and calcium, both known to help reduce blood pressure.

Meal 3 (lunch salad with a protein)

1½ cups of mixture of romaine and spinach or kale

6—8 oz. cod, grilled, baked or however you like it

1 tablespoon balsamic vinaigrette or other low fat, low calorie dressing

¼ cup chopped pecans or almonds

NAKED Tip

Here's a salad dressing one of my closest friends loves on her "NAKED" salads: 2 tablespoons sesame oil, 2 tablespoons rice vinegar, 2 tablespoons crushed almonds or pecans (very well crushed!). Since the proportions are even, you can increase or decrease to your liking and even drizzle a bit of this on your cod. I like to create my salad and then place my fish or poultry on top.

Meal 4 (snack)

½ cup dried prunes and raisins mix

NAKED Tip

Prunes are a great source of energy and high in fiber, vitamins and minerals. Raisins are simply dehydrated grapes, also rich in nutrients and a great source of B vitamins, iron and potassium. And they too are a great source of energy.

NAKED Tip

The snack options in this book are not widely varied, and that is intentional to keep the menu very simple and you focused. Dr. Oz, for example, has spoken publicly many times about how his diet is quite narrow and he only switches things up occasionally to reinvigorate his taste buds.

Meal 5 (dinner)

6—8 oz. of salmon, chicken or lean turkey

Small side salad (e.g. 1 cup or less of spinach or kale) with chopped tomatoes and dressing.

NAKED Tip

A great seasoning for fish and meats is called "Greek seasoning" and you can get it at Penzys.com. It's a mixture of lemon, garlic and oregano, and I have sprinkled it on many of my lunch and dinner proteins.

Meal 6 (optional, can replace another meal or be a snack)

¼ cup of nuts
½ cup of berries
or
1 cup of popcorn, air popped and no butter, okay to season with a tbsp. herbs or spices
½ cup of berries
or
1 rice cake with 1 tbsp. of raw peanut butter or almond butter
¼ cup of berries

NAKED Tip

Green apples are rich in vitamin C and very fibrous. They are also one of the best snacks for helping fight heart disease and diabetes.

Mind/Spirit Tip: Apologize to the People You've Hurt

In the last chapter I talked about the importance of showing gratitude. Something even more beneficial, in my experience, is when you reach out to the people you've hurt and apologize. Live long enough, and your unresolved burdens become something you can feel. It weighs on your shoulders like an overstuffed backpack. A simple face-to-face apology can relieve that burden in an instant. It's one of the most freeing feelings in the world.

One summer, I wholeheartedly dedicated myself to this idea. At the time there were about 12 people—ex-husbands, ex-boyfriends, ex-friends—who I'd hurt but who had never heard me say "I'm sorry." Each of these broken relationships was weighing me down. So I tracked them down one by one. Some lived closer to me than others. One man lived nine hours away by car. I picked a day, started driving and made a weekend out of it. (Looking back, I probably could have flown.)

By the end of the summer, I'd met face-to-face with all of them. For me, the emotions were still raw when I knocked on each door, not knowing what to expect on the other side. How could I know how each of them felt toward me after the way things ended? I didn't care. I had no fear. One man stood there in silence after I said my peace, perplexed. "I meant every word of it, and I hope you have a great week," I told him, then turned around. He said nothing as I walked away, and that was okay. We hadn't seen each other in a while, and he probably didn't know how to comprehend it all. I'd like to think he truly thought about everything I said the rest of that day. In the end, it doesn't matter. I knew I would feel better for apologizing, and I did.

Can you feel the same peace without apologizing in person? Maybe, but your emotions don't always translate via email, text or phone call. Your tone of voice can say a lot. So does the look in your eyes. It means more to the other person to actually hear an apology face-to-face. And sometimes, it blows their mind.

If you've ever been involved in a 12-step program, you know that apologizing to the people you've hurt is one of the recommended steps to recovery. But you don't have to be a recovering addict to feel the burden of an unresolved relationship. A guilty conscience can weigh on any of us. During my Summer Apology Tour, my guiding thought was that if I died tomorrow, I could rest knowing I'd made peace with everyone I'd wronged.

Some people simply have a difficult time apologizing. If that's you, and you've read this far, you have no excuse not to learn this critical skill. Here's how to do it in three steps, according to an essay psychologist Guy Winch wrote for Psychology Today:

1. Make a statement of regret for what happened.
2. Make a clear 'I'm sorry' statement.
3. Make a request for forgiveness.

These ingredients must be delivered with sincerity for an apology to be effective. You can't fake sincerity, so don't apologize until you're ready. Then again, don't hold onto your apology so long that it's weighing on you physically. And if you drive nine hours to unload that weight, the person you're apologizing to probably won't question your sincerity.

Day Nine

"All our dreams can come true if we have the courage to pursue them."
—Walt Disney

Today you will follow the same upper body weight-training workout you did on Day Two. The focus will be on your shoulders, back and arms.

Feel free to swap out some of the exercises for a particular body part with any of the ones listed on Day One, but continue to follow proper technique and the proper amount of reps. The reason for this is that some of you may work out in a gym and some of you may work out at home; some of you may have dumbbells and some of you many have resistance bands. The circuit is designed to give you a base to follow but variations can and should happen so you can get the most out of your muscles and prevent boredom.

Drink plenty of fluids throughout this workout, and make sure you drink after as well.

Before you begin your workout, remember to warm up the upper body with the **shoulder and arm warm-up**, and be sure to follow the proper form so you are getting the most out of your workout.

Circuit 1 (shoulder blast) standing or seated
Dumbbell (DB) front raise 12—15 reps
Side lateral seated DB raises 12—15 reps
Seated DB presses 12—15 reps
DB upright rows 12—15 reps
Repeat circuit three to five times
Rest period 30—45 seconds

Circuit 2 (back and arms)

Tricep high lateral rope pull-downs12—15 reps
Speed rows using band in squatting position 30—45 seconds
Tricep push-downs on cable machine 15—20 reps
Standing DB curls 12—15 reps
Repeat circuit three to five times
Rest period 30—45 seconds

Circuit 3

One-arm DB row on flat bench 12—15 reps
Tricep kickbacks using DB 15—20 reps
Seated concentration DB curls 15—20 each arm
Repeat three to five times
Rest period 30—45 seconds

Circuit 4

Seated cable rows (machine) 12—15 reps
Standing tricep push-downs using tubing or bands 12—15 reps
Standing bicep curls 12—15 reps
Repeat three to five times
Rest period 30—45 seconds

At the end of your upper body workout, proceed to the abdominal circuit.

NAKED Tip

Lift enough weight to make it worthwhile. You'll know you have the right set of weights when your muscles feel fatigued after three sets of about eight to 12 reps. Don't be married to this size dumbbell. Respond to your stronger muscles by gradually increasing the weight you lift over time.

NAKED Tip

Don't rush through your reps. If you move too quickly you're not only at risk for an injury, but you're also more likely to rely on momentum to offset, which translates to not using your muscles. Move slowly and with control to ensure you're targeting the intended areas.

NAKED Tip

Sports drinks are tempting and can give you a boost, but they are also high in sugar and calories. Stay hydrated with water before, during and after your workout for better results and performance.

Meal 1 (pre-workout)

Protein smoothie

1 scoop of protein powder shaken with 8 oz. of water.

Meal 2 (post-workout)

2 whole eggs, 1 egg white (cage free), 1 oz. baby spinach, 1 tsp coconut oil to make omelet; 1/8 tsp sea salt

¼ avocado

NAKED Tip

Yesterday I mentioned some health benefits of green apples. There are many more, but one important one is that they help you lose weight because of the high fiber content. They help you feel full and also help speed up your metabolism. So try to introduce green apples into your daily routine early in the day to get a good high-energy start.

Meal 3 (lunch salad with a protein)

1½ cup mixed greens, spinach, baby spinach, baby kale, or a mix of both

6—8 oz. of lean meat

¼ cup of slivered almonds

1 tbsp. of dressing

NAKED Tip

Speaking of green apples, another great way to integrate them is to chop them up into little chunks and mix them in with your salad. They go especially well with chopped walnuts.

Meal 4 (snack)

1 hard-boiled egg

NAKED Tip

I make a dozen hard-boiled eggs on Sunday for the week ahead and reach for them through the week. Hard-boiled eggs are a protein that help satisfy hunger and give you fuel to burn.

Meal 5 (dinner)

6—8 oz. Tilapia

Small side salad (e.g. 1 cup or less of spinach or kale) with chopped tomatoes and dressing

½ cup black beans alone or sprinkled on your salad

NAKED Tip

Beans are packed with fiber and literally fill you up. They are the ultimate weight-loss food!

Meal 6 (optional, can replace another meal or be a snack)

¼ cup of nuts

½ cup of berries

or

1 cup of popcorn, no butter, okay to season with a tbsp. herbs or spices

½ cup of berries

or

1 rice cake with 1 tbsp. of raw peanut butter or almond butter

¼ cup of berries

NAKED Tip

Yoga! Did you know yoga stimulates the vagus nerve, a nerve that runs from your brainstem to your abdomen and acts as a superhighway to bring vital information to and from the brain? The vagus nerve is responsible for your entire digestive system, breathing and heart rate. And this is why there are so many health benefits to yoga. A great way to start or end any day is with a bit of yoga. There are many videos on demand and on YouTube that you can access to tap into a nice yoga routine.

Mind/Spirit Tip: Don't Let Your Pride Get in the Way

Many years ago, I had a business partner with whom I ran a gym. She ran into trouble when her life got in the way of work, which happens to all of us at times. Her marriage was falling apart and she was running out of money, some of which we needed to run the company. With the world bearing down on her, she broke down and confessed.

"I don't think I can go forward anymore," she said. "I'm probably going to get divorced."

I was shocked at first, but confession is good for the soul, and I respected her for being vulnerable with me. "I'm sorry this is happening to you," I said. "We'll ride the rough waters together. It's going to be okay."

It was a good conversation for both of us. Too bad it never happened.

Unfortunately I can only imagine how much easier it would have been for me, and how much better it would have been for our company, if she had said those words that day. Instead, her solution was to leave the company cold and take half the inventory telling me why. I lost my business partner and my best friend that day. It felt like a divorce.

The Bible says pride goes before destruction, and I've seen it for myself. If my partner hadn't allowed her pride to get in the way, she might have been blown away by the acceptance she felt after confessing what was going on in her personal life. Pride can be a huge impediment to our mental and spiritual health, not to mention our personal and professional lives.

Psychology tells us there are two types of pride. You can conveniently think of them as good pride and bad pride; the technical terms are "*authentic pride*" and "*hubristic pride*." Authentic pride is closely related to the traits of genuine self-esteem (like authenticity), while hubristic pride is similar to the traits of narcissistic self-aggrandizement (such as perceiving social consensus—the notion that everyone around you shares the same beliefs as one another). People with hubristic pride were more likely to feel arrogance and egotism, be socially uncomfortable, anxious about relationships and insecure about being liked. People with authentic pride were less sensitive to rejection.

It's okay to take pride in who you are and what you've accomplished. In fact, I couldn't endorse it more. The question is, which kind of pride are you really feeling? The difference between good and bad pride is as different as night and day. If you attribute your success to something stable and controllable, like effort, you're probably feeling authentic pride. People with authentic pride understand a marriage can fail despite their best efforts. A divorce doesn't have to affect the pride you take in your work, if you can accept the parts that are your fault and move on. Confessing you've lost control over an uncontrollable situation shouldn't be a stumbling block to your ego.

More than how much pride you have, it's what you do with it that counts. There are times you'll want to let it shine, like in a job interview. Other times, you'll need to set it aside and apologize to someone, ask another person for help or confess something you're not particularly proud about. As you get closer in touch with your naked mind and spirit, think about the role pride plays in your life. Can you set it aside when you need to?

Day Ten

"What seems to us as bitter trials are often blessings in disguise."
—Oscar Wilde

Today you are back to doing your cardio and abs workout. Do your stretching and warm-up activity and stay hydrated.

I've discussed the many benefits of cardio exercise throughout this book, but some of the benefits go far beyond weight loss. Researchers all across the globe found heart- and sweat-pumping cardio exercises are not only good for your overall health but have positive effects on your memory and learning, something we all need to pay close attention to as we age.

Continue to increase the amount of cardio you are doing and think about the long-term benefits it will bring to your life as you continue on this journey.

NAKED Tip

If you are running on a treadmill, let go of the handrail. Holding onto the side of the treadmill does more harm than good. Gripping the rails decreases energy output and oxygen consumption, significantly reducing the effectiveness of a workout. Go hands free then pump your arms from waist to chest, not across the body (which can slow you down).

NAKED Tip

Need more motivation while running? Forgo the fancy fitness gadgets and crank up the tunes. Listening to music during exercise has been shown to improve performance, increase motivation and put distractions (like negative thoughts and fatigue) at bay.

NAKED Tip

Build a workout routine around team sports, group activities, or fitness classes to boost performance during cardio exercise. It can make the entire gym experience more enjoyable, with a built-in boost of accountability.

Meal 1 (pre-workout)

Protein smoothie

1 scoop of protein powder shaken with 8 oz. of water.

NAKED Tip

"Fast carbs" are carbs that enter the bloodstream quickly and therefore raise your blood sugar levels. Your body needs some carbs to give you energy, but you want those that enter the bloodstream slowly. The carbohydrates I highlight in the NAKED Program, such as beans and berries, are in the slow carb category and provide important sources of energy.

Meal 2 (post-workout)

2 whole eggs, 1 egg white (cage free), 1 oz. baby spinach, 1 tsp coconut oil to make omelet; ⅛ tsp sea salt

NAKED Tip

Many people like to mix flaxseed in smoothies, sprinkle it in salads, or even scramble it with eggs. Flaxseeds help lower cholesterol because they are a natural source of Omega-3 fats. They also contain lots of B vitamins.

Meal 3 (lunch salad with a protein)

1 can of white tuna in water

1 cup mix of chopped broccoli, cauliflower, red onion and celery

Mix ¼ cup of olive oil with 3 tablespoons lemon juice, 2 tablespoons soy sauce, 1 tsp mustard.

<u>NAKED Tip</u>

Warm liquids help wake up the intestines to promote bowel movements. And yes, regular bowel movements are very important to your overall health. A cup of coffee or tea in the morning is a good thing!

Meal 4 (snack)

1 cup of homemade slaw. Combine a carrot, turnip, beet, and cup of cabbage in a grater. Add some diced onion and an oil and vinegar dressing, toss and enjoy.

<u>NAKED Tip</u>

The slaw I've made here above is a fat burner. Make more and enjoy it as a snack throughout the week. Also, I chose a vinegar dressing because vinegar naturally helps lower potassium levels if your potassium levels are high. Generally speaking, high potassium levels are bad for the kidneys but also cause the muscles to break down.

Meal 5 (dinner)

6—8 oz. lean turkey or chicken

1 cup of boiled broccoli, Brussels sprouts or cauliflower

<u>NAKED Tip</u>

Asparagus is a great vegetable you can add to any meal. It is loaded with fiber and also a great anti-inflammatory.

Meal 6 (optional, can replace another meal or be a snack)

¼ cup of nuts

½ cup of berries

or

1 cup of popcorn, no butter, okay to season with a tbsp. herbs or spices

½ cup of berries

or

1 rice cake with 1 tbsp. of raw peanut butter or almond butter

¼ cup of berries

NAKED Tip

Cranberries and strawberries are rich in quercetin, which has a strong anti-inflammatory effect on the body.

Mind/Spirit Tip: Respect Others

This goes without saying, right? Reap what you sow, and others will plant good seeds back into your heart.

Now more than ever, all of us need to be intentional about giving others respect. It benefits the people around you in the moment, and it benefits you in the long run. Remember, your spirit isn't just something that guides your own awareness of the world, it's something by which others judge you. Your spirit will either attract or repel the people around you, so project a spirit of respect.

We all want to be respected, and we all feel disrespected at times. That's nothing new. Only there is something new in our society: we see disrespect everywhere, to the point of being tolerated—even expected—in some arenas. Take something big, like a presidential election. The moderator of one 2015 presidential debate said in closing, "We also appreciate your helping save time by talking over one another at times." That backhanded compliment was offered to a group of people who believe they're qualified to lead the United States of America. The behavior of our leaders has a way of trickling down to the rest of society. Think about your Facebook friends-turned-political-experts. Is the tone of their debates respectful?

Political causes tend to bring out our fiery side, so maybe occasional bickering isn't so surprising. Yet we see basic respect missing elsewhere in our daily lives. One of my colleagues recently sent an email asking three questions. The person responded by answering one of the questions and ignoring the other two. Was this an "oversight" or a symptom of living in a world whose means of communication are endless?

In Day 25, I explain the broad dangers of smartphone overuse. The implications extend to basic respect. In her book *Unfettered Hope: A Call to Faithful Living in an Affluent Society*, author Marva J. Dawn explains that "technology has... moved beyond its proper vocation to create an orientation that has shifted away from engagement in practices that relate to what is most important to us. Instead, society is characterized by the proliferation of devices that produces an endless stream of commodities unrelated to any context and thereby leaving consumers without a world of relationships."

That's a long and fancy way of saying that as a society, we aren't very good at relating to each other anymore. One by-product, I think, is a decrease in respect. Computers, tablets and smartphones have enabled almost limitless communication—emails, text messages, Facebook posts, snapchats and tweets. These are all so informal now, it's almost embarrassing. We would be naive to think this doesn't affect our face--to--face interactions too.

The scary part is what this means for future generations. People my age can still remember when the sound of a ringing phone brought excitement and anticipation of who might be calling, or when almost every written communication began with the word "*dear*." My grandchildren won't have these memories. While I recognize the convenience we've gained through technology, I also recognize what we've lost. It's better to show too much respect than not enough. We'd all rather have someone over--respect us than not respect us at all.

Next time you have the choice, why not pick up the phone, place a good old-fashioned phone call and listen to someone else's voice? It's only a little less convenient than a text message and it allows us to relate a little more closely to each other. That's a sign of respect in and of itself!

Day Eleven

"I am determined to be cheerful and happy in whatever situation I may find myself. For I have learned that the greater part of our misery or unhappiness is determined not by our circumstance but by our disposition."

—Martha Washington

Today you will follow the same lower body weight-training workout you did on Day Four. The focus will be on your legs and buttocks. Be sure to begin with the hamstring glute stretch to get your muscles warmed up and ready to go.

Strong glutes ensure you keep proper form during weight training, especially lower body exercises, so your knees are protected. It also protects you from injury, improves athletic performance and gives you that sexy, curvy shape we all aspire to.

Feel free to swap out or add in any of the exercises for the legs and glutes from the list of exercises in Chapter Three. If you're a beginner, swap out standard squats for jump squats for a high performance workout. Do as many jump squats as you can and finish up with standard squats.

Drink plenty of water and don't forget to complete your workout with the abdominal circuit.

Lower body circuit (45 to 60 minutes)

Five-minute warm-up

Leg extensions, 15—20 reps, four sets

Circuit 1

Smith machine squats, 15—20 reps
Walking lunges, 50—75 yards
Seated or kneeling leg curls machine, 15—20 reps
Repeat three or four sets
Rest period 30—45 seconds

Circuit 2

Seated leg press (machine) 15—20 reps
Standing body weight squats 30—40 reps
Anterior reach lunge 12—15 each leg
Repeat four to five times
Rest period 30—45 seconds

Circuit 3

Jump squats 30 sec
Alternating jumping lunges 30 sec
Repeat three to four times
Rest period 30—45 seconds

Circuit 4

Lying glute bridge off stability ball, legs straight 15—20 reps
Lying glute bridge with knees bent, feet flat on ball, pushing hips up as high as you can 15—20 reps
Lying leg curls on stability ball 15—20 reps
Repeat three to four times
Rest period 30—45 seconds

<u>NAKED Tip</u>

For a variation on traditional squats, try wall squats. This is one of the exercises that strengthens the quadriceps muscles, which are some of the largest muscles in your body. This workout also benefits your buttocks. Strengthening these muscles will help you rise from a chair quickly and climb stairs easily.

<u>NAKED Tip</u>

Having a strong lower body will help develop better balance, which is essential, especially as you age. Exercises like side lunges and deadlifts will increase your stability and help keep you ready for anything. Whether you're a performance junkie or a weekend-warrior type, balance is essential for maintaining control of your body.

NAKED Tip

Strength training will not only make you stronger, but it can speed up your metabolism and burn more calories. It's no secret that lifting weights helps people build and maintain muscle mass. And when your body composition has more muscle, your whole body works more efficiently. Strength training outperforms standard cardio exercises when it comes to increasing metabolism.

Meal 1 (pre-workout)

Protein smoothie

1 scoop of protein powder shaken with 8 oz. of water.

NAKED Tip

As you exercise more, you are also losing more water through sweat, which means you need to drink more water. Water increases your physical performance, gives you more energy and helps your digestive tract work efficiently. Water also increases brain function, allows you to concentrate and even stay in a better mood!

Meal 2 (post-workout)

2 eggs and 1 egg white (cage free), scrambled or as an omelet

¼ cup chopped onion

¼ cup tomatoes

NAKED Tip

I like to scramble my eggs with onions to give them flavor. Consider the eggs as your base and add what you like to make it tasty.

Meal 3 (lunch salad with a protein)

6—8 oz. flank steak steak, pan-grilled or seared

1½ cup mixed greens, spinach, baby spinach, baby kale, or a mix of both

¼ cup of slivered almonds

1 tbsp. of dressing

1 avocado

NAKED Tip

Flank steak is a lean beef filled with vitamin B12, which aids in red blood cell production, and iron, also good for those red blood cells and carrying oxygen throughout the body.

NAKED Tip

Adding an avocado to your lunch salad will give it an extra kick of flavor and also pairs with lean beef.

Meal 4 (snack)

1 rice cake with raw peanut butter or raw almond butter
or
¼ cup almonds or walnuts

NAKED Tip

You can also make an avocado a snack. Avocados are also high in protein and fiber.

Meal 5 (dinner)

6—8 oz. cod
1½ cup baby kale or mixed greens
1 cup chopped tomatoes
Salt and pepper to taste

NAKED Tip

You may have noticed I have a tomato with nearly all salads. That's because I love them and also because they are loaded with health benefits. Tomatoes contain large amounts of lycopene, a powerful antioxidant that helps prevent cell damage. Lycopene is also the natural chemical that causes certain fruits and vegetables to be red.

Meal 6 (optional, can replace another meal or be a snack)

¼ cup of nuts
½ cup of berries
or
1—2 cups of popcorn, no butter, okay to season with a tbsp. herbs or spices
½ cup of berries

or
1 rice cake with 1 tbsp. of raw peanut butter or almond butter
¼ cup of berries

NAKED Tip

The lowest calorie nuts are almonds, followed by cashews and pistachios. You can always grab about ¼ cup of nuts as an afternoon snack and always choose raw or dry roasted.

Mind/Spirit Tip: Forgive Freely

I can still remember the first time something was stolen from me. This was my most prized possession in the world at the time, so to get it back I contacted the most skilled police officer I knew. She delivered. Before I knew it, my mom had found my doll and returned it to its rightful owner. My sister was the culprit. I forgave her.

As you grow older, you'll lose things more valuable than a childhood toy: friends, your virginity, your faith in other people. Some of these things might be lost forever. They can be stolen at ordinary moments that suddenly become extraordinary for their deep sense of loss. When someone wrongs you, it can be a traumatic spiritual setback. Responding to such a setback is a challenge you'll be called to at some point.

And let's face it: being robbed is brutal. Often, the feeling you'll never get something back is more damaging than the actual loss. Material goods can be replaced; a friend, for example, cannot. When somebody especially close to you betrays your trust, it can feel like a death in the family. Sometimes that's essentially what it becomes, if the relationship dies entirely.

It's okay to mourn your losses. Necessary, even. But when people steal from us, we must make a conscious effort not to become jaded or hardened. Building boundaries between ourselves and others is the "safe" thing to do. It's our instinct. It takes a bigger person not to lose your sense of compassion, not to let being robbed overcome you, overtake you and change who you are.

After having something valuable stolen from my home as an adult, I had a choice: forgive and move on, or withdraw out of the fear of being robbed again. The choice was easy. After everything I'd been through, I wasn't about to quit inviting guests into my home to see my beautiful closet for charity fundraisers. This, I felt, was a wonderful thing I could do for God—at the exact time when Satan usually chases us in earnest.

Even after my sister stole my favorite doll, I was quick to see the good in everyone. My biggest challenge was accepting that evil exists in the world. This fact is unavoidable every time we're robbed. Rather than dwelling on our losses, let's mourn, then forgive, then learn, then grow as human beings.

Remember the World's Happiest Man (Day Three)? He once allowed an American neuroscientist to wire 256 sensors to his skull at the University of Wisconsin. He was meditating on compassion when the sensors recorded record levels of gamma waves, which are linked to consciousness, attention, learning and memory. Literally, the professor said, existing literature on neuroscience had never seen anything like it.

So, compassion doesn't just benefit the recipient. It benefits you in ways you can't imagine. This book isn't just about being physically naked. It's about being emotionally naked too. You can't be emotionally naked if you're holding onto a burden. Consider too that you will need to forgive yourself at times—if you eat something you shouldn't, or skip a day of working out. Take a look in the mirror and tell yourself, "It's okay. Just get back on track tomorrow." After all, no one is perfect. We all make mistakes. Even perfect schedules fall apart periodically.

When you don't forgive, you merely hang on to your hurt and give it a chance to consume you. Only by forgiving can you let that hurt go. We might never forget the wrong others inflict upon us, but we can always forgive.

Day Twelve

"People hate cardio. I hate cardio. But pick the top five songs that you love. Do your cardio during these songs, and you're done. I'd say 95 percent of the time you don't even know you just did it."

—Taylor Kitch

You all know what today is.

Follow your workout with the abs series and increase your reps. Do your stretching and drink your water.

Make a good playlist.

NAKED Tip

Hop on the treadmill, crank up the speed, and don't forget to adjust the incline. As the incline increases, so will your heart rate, sending the calorie burn through the roof. Bumping up the incline to a 5.5 percent grade or higher can also strengthen the legs and core, not to mention improve running form and sprint speed.

NAKED Tip

Research suggests that working out first thing in the morning is best for creating and sticking to the habit of exercising. However, not everyone is a morning person. Don't get hung up on that. The good news is the body will adapt to training at any point in the day, as long as it is done on a consistent basis.

NAKED Tip

For a non-impact alternative to running and other cardio workouts, try swimming. Swimming is great because it provides a full-body cardio workout that will burn hundreds of calories per hour. To ensure your muscles get pushed to the limit by this form of cardio, alternate between the different stroke styles, moving from breaststroke to front stroke to backstroke. This will ensure you target all the muscles in the body from a variety of angles to maximize your workout.

Meal 1 (pre-workout)

Protein smoothie

1 scoop of protein powder shaken with 8 oz. of water.

NAKED Tip

Add ½ cup of oats to your protein shake for a delicious boost.

Meal 2 (post-workout)

2 eggs, 1 egg white (cage-free) for scrambled eggs or omelet with:

¼ cup chopped red onion

½ chopped green pepper

⅓ cup spinach

NAKED Tip

Try a delicious egg in a hole: Take 1 large acorn squash, cut it in half, and level off the bottoms so they can sit on a baking pan, scoop out seeds and membrane, spray with olive oil, season with salt and pepper or your favorite seasonings, and bake for about 20 minutes. Add an egg to the center and place back in the oven for about 15 minutes or until the egg is cooked to taste. This recipe makes two so you have one to share, or you can just make one and save the other half for later.

Meal 3 (lunch salad with a protein)

6—8 oz. grilled skinless chicken breast or lean turkey

1½ cup mixed greens, spinach, baby spinach, baby kale, or a mix of both

1 chopped tomato

¼ cup of slivered almonds

1 tbsp. of dressing

NAKED Tip

For another great salad, consider tossing in some beets and walnuts with spinach or kale.

Meal 4 (snack)

Rice cake with mashed banana spread.

NAKED Tip

Many fans have written to me that they like the plain rice cakes with tuna on top as a snack. Sprinkle this with well-chopped celery to give it even more crunch.

Meal 5 (dinner)

6—8 oz. grilled skinless chicken breasts, sliced into strips
1 or 2 cups mixed greens
¼ red onion, sliced in long, thin slices
½ cup black beans
1 tablespoon dressing

NAKED Tip

If you had a red meat for lunch, go for a leaner option like fish at dinner. You also may find that with so many meals, you're just plain full. Don't over eat, but remember you need fuel for that fire to burn off the fat!

Meal 6 (optional, can replace another meal or be a snack)

¼ cup of nuts
½ cup of berries
or
1 cup of popcorn, no butter, okay to season with a tbsp. herbs or spices
½ cup of berries
or
1 rice cake with 1 tbsp. of raw peanut butter or almond butter
¼ cup of berries

NAKED Tip

A fan wrote to me that he tosses a tablespoon or two of Old Bay

Seasoning with his popcorn to give it a kick. You might try this, or even red pepper if you like spicy foods.

Mind/Spirit Tip: Take Ownership of Your Wellbeing

Imagine you've hired someone to clean your house. They're dusting and vacuuming and moving furniture around to get everything clean. What would you do if they forgot to put something back in its place—a lamp, a chair, a vase? Would you leave it where it is, or move it back where you want it?

Taking ownership of your body shouldn't be any different. If your body doesn't look the way you want it to, don't just stand there making excuses for why it looks the way it does. Do something! When I talk to women my age and older who want to get into shape, I can always count on hearing excuses for why they're overweight. They may hate how they look and feel, but every single one of them has an excuse. I've heard them all. "I don't have cartilage in my knees." "My back is bad." They all want a shortcut around the excuse, a magic remedy for how to lose weight without working out.

The truth is, I've trained women and men in wheelchairs. I've trained people who can't move without a walker, who have no way to get down to a floor mat. (We did our workout on a table). No cartilage in your knees, your shoulders, your elbows? No problem. I've worked with clients whose arthritis was so bad, they couldn't comb their hair on their own. What did they all have in common? The determination to better their health. They were willing to take ownership of their wellbeing in spite of the excuses.

If you feel like you've hit a wall and you're ready to give in to an excuse, here's my advice: watch the Paralympic Games. (They have their own YouTube channel if they aren't on TV.) If someone without legs can play hockey, or someone without arms can swim, what's your excuse today? If you have no knees, find a health club with a rowing machine. If you have joint problems, hop in a pool. You'll be weightless.

Maybe your excuse isn't physical. If you're human, you've probably made commitments to your family and/or your career that compete with the time you set aside to take care of yourself. I get it. Those commitments can really add up. In the moment, it might be hard to view the way we look and feel as the sum of our own choices. But taking ownership of your wellbeing means taking responsibility for the consequences of your actions. Maybe you didn't need to stay up late watching TV with the family—next time, maybe you can ride a bike with your kids during the daytime instead.

If you do have a physical disability, you have options. Certified personal trainers are typically trained in adaptive fitness techniques. Many gyms have adaptive equipment. Train with the right person in the right setting and they can get you started on the right path, to the point where you're able to train on your own. I've been living with back problems for years. Working out hardly cures my pain—it hurts—but I can't let it become an excuse to let my body fall apart. When in pain, look for the things you can do and don't dwell on the things you can't.

It's essential to your mind and spirit that you take ownership for how you look and feel physically. Otherwise, you'll just be consumed by excuses. To change your life in any way, it all starts with you doing the work.

Day Thirteen

"If you are going through hell, keep going."
—Winston S. Churchill

This is your last workout day of the second week of my program. We return to the upper body series of exercises targeting the chest, shoulders and back. You will recognize the strength training circuit from Day Five. Push yourself to increase your reps if your body feels ready to do so.

Increase your range of motion during your pushups by lowering your body closer to the ground, and if you are a beginner, do one more push-up without using your knees. Once again, you may feel free to swap out the existing exercises for any of the body parts you are working out today with any of the exercises mentioned in Chapter Three.

Do your **shoulder and arm warm-up**. Drink plenty of water, and don't forget to complete your workout with the abdominal circuit.

Circuit 1 (back)

Lat pull-downs, three sets of 15 reps
Seated rows, three sets of 15 reps
Assisted pull-ups, three sets of 15 reps
Repeat three to five times
Rest period, 30—45 seconds

Circuit 2 (chest)

Standard push-ups, 20 reps
Dumbbell presses, three sets of 15
Reverse push-ups on the resistance ball
Repeat three to five times
Rest period 30—45 seconds

Circuit 3 (shoulders)

Dumbbell (DB) front raise, 12—15 reps
Side lateral seated DB raises, 12—15 reps
Seated DB presses, 12—15 reps
DB upright rows, 12—15 reps
Repeat circuit three to five times
Rest period, 30—45 seconds

NAKED Tip

Having strong shoulders can help to improve your posture, but that's not the only benefit. When you combine shoulder-strengthening exercises with shoulder stretches, it also gives you the strength and flexibility to easily perform everyday tasks. Having strong shoulders can also help prevent injuries to the rotator cuff.

NAKED Tip

Push-ups help improve muscular balance, which is important in building up strength, and you can do them almost anywhere—at the gym, at home or at your office. They can be done with just your body weight, or you can add supplemental weight on your back, change your hand position or create an unstable surface in order to increase the challenge. You can also do pushups on a decline—elevating your feet above your heart—to make this already challenging exercise even harder. The height of the elevation of your feet during the exercise makes a difference. The higher your feet are, the more challenging the pushup will be.

NAKED Tip

Pull-ups act as a great toning workout for the upper body. Don't belong to a gym or can't make it there? Consider purchasing an over-the-doorway pull-up bar for your home. They are inexpensive and easy to install.

Meal 1 (pre-workout)

Protein smoothie
1 scoop of protein powder shaken with 8 oz. of water.

NAKED Tip:

Add ¼ cup of finely ground nuts and seeds to your smoothie to give it some texture. Suggested nuts: almonds, walnuts, sesame seeds or sunflower seeds.

Meal 2 (post-workout)

¼ cup cream of rice cereal mixed in 1 cup of water

Boil the rice/water mixture in the microwave for about three minutes.

1 tsp of cinnamon sprinkled on top and/or a pinch of sea salt

NAKED Tip

Alternate snacks include: ¼ cup of raw or roasted almonds (no salt!), ¼ cup of walnuts, ¼ cup of berries or 1 apple.

Meal 3 (lunch salad with a protein)

1½ cup mixed greens, spinach, baby spinach, baby kale, or a mix of both

6—8 oz. of lean meat

¼ cup of slivered almonds

1 tbsp. of dressing

NAKED Tip

There are so many ways to blend a nice vinaigrette. Olive oil can be mixed with nearly any type of vinegar, including white, cider and wine vinegar. Add black pepper and sea salt to taste.

Meal 4 (snack)

1 rice cake with 1 tbsp. raw peanut butter or raw almond butter spread on top.

NAKED Tip

If you like spicy foods, try a plain rice cake sprinkled with red pepper and sea salt to taste.

Meal 5 (dinner)

6—8 oz. of salmon

Small side salad (i.e. 1 cup or less of spinach or kale) with chopped tomatoes and dressing

NAKED Tip

Always buy wild caught salmon and never farm-raised salmon. Farmed salmon contain pesticides and other harmful chemicals. Choose salmon specifically labeled wild, Alaskan or Chinook.

Meal 6 (optional, can replace another meal or be a snack)

¼ cup of nuts

½ cup of berries

or

1 cup of popcorn, air popped and no butter, okay to season with a tbsp. herbs or spices

½ cup of berries

or

1 rice cake with 1 tbsp. of raw peanut butter or almond butter

¼ cup of berries

NAKED Tip

Every once in a while when you have a sweet tooth, you might want to grab for some chocolate. Go for dark chocolate, which has natural anti-inflammatory properties. Chocolate contains a saturated fat called stearic acid, but this type of fat does not raise cholesterol levels. A small piece of chocolate with high percentages of cocoa, no more than three times per week, can actually protect your heart.

Mind/Spirit Tip: Don't Give in to Excuses

Apollo Creed had a famous line in the movie *Rocky III*. "When we fought," Apollo told Rocky, "you had that eye of the tiger, man; the edge! And now you gotta get it back." Legend has it the band Survivor heard that line when they screened the film, then wrote the song- "Eye of the Tiger"—to fit the movie. The song became more than just a theme to a famous film. It's an anthem for perseverance.

Full confession: "Eye of the Tiger" is my song. When I'm trying to push through a challenge, Survivor starts to play in my head. Those are the words I summon when the odds are against me. If you're stuck in a cubicle on a weekday afternoon and truly, mentally stuck, go ahead and start humming those famous power chords. Get the "Eye of the Tiger" by whatever means necessary, however corny it might seem.

In 2014, *Fortune* magazine asked 40 of the world's most prominent business leaders to share their best advice for success. Harold M.

Messmer, the CEO of Robert Half International and one of the richest Americans alive, cited *The Little Engine That Could,* a children's book about a train, as a source of inspiration for his own perseverance.

Excuses to back down from a challenge are always easy to find. You won't need 30 days to find one. They're everywhere. All the time. It's much harder to find a reason to push through a massive obstacle—but it's extremely important to your mental and spiritual wellbeing that you do it. Otherwise, how will we ever know what we're capable of accomplishing?

Persistence always starts in your mind but extends naturally to your body. While climbing Mt. Kilimanjaro, the highest peak in Africa, I was attacked by a parasite and fell ill. Still, only a stretcher could pull me down from that mountain. I'd committed to summiting the mountain for a charity organization, Child Legacy International. Nineteen thousand feet later and still sick as a dog, I realized I wouldn't need that stretcher. I had reached the top. Try telling my donors, or my children, it wasn't important to push through those obstacles (even though medically I was near death).

What does "pushing through" mean, exactly? For me, it's a little voice inside my head that says, "You still haven't given 150 percent." If I throw in the towel, I need to be able to say I gave nothing less than my best. At least then I can go to sleep knowing it wasn't possible to exert any more effort, to try any harder, than I did.

So, how good *can* you look naked? The answer to that question will require some stubbornness on your part, but stubbornness can be a rewarding virtue. Being stubborn doesn't mean being stupid. Mixed with just the right amount of wisdom, a little stubbornness can be a powerful thing. In business, for example, it's especially wise to have a Plan B, C and D mapped out just in case Plan A falls through. Always give 150 percent toward Plan A. But if that plan isn't meant to be for whatever reason, at least you'll have a fallback.

Other times, straying off course isn't an option. It's your time. Maybe you have children who are in college or high school. Of course, you would never tell them to let one class, one professor or one bad semester stand in the way of graduating or getting the grades they want. If you can talk the talk, walk the walk: Your own 30-day journey can set an example for your family.

Find the Eye of the Tiger. Find the voice of perseverance that speaks to you.

Day Fourteen

"Muscles are torn in the gym, fed in the kitchen and built in bed."
—Gymface.com

Welcome to your rest day! You have now completed two weeks of my NAKED Program. You are well on your way to a healthy new you. Take some time today to relish what you have already accomplished.

When you exercise you tear muscle fibers. Without rest days you are unable to give your muscles a chance to grow and repair. Remember to get plenty of sleep, drink lots of water, and eat healthy. Take care of your body, and it will take care of you!

<u>NAKED Tip</u>

Although massages can be costly, they are a great way to relax. They are particularly enjoyable and beneficial after a good workout, and I just love them. There are many benefits to getting a massage. They improve flexibility, aid with muscle recovery, help to increase your range of motion and of course they make you feel fabulous! If cost is an issue, research spa and massage chains in your area. Most have inexpensive rates and special deals.

<u>NAKED Tip</u>

The National Heart, Lung and Blood Institute recommends at least seven to eight hours of sleep a night for adults. Sleep is essential for muscle repair and to restore your body's energy. Here are a few tips for getting a good night's sleep: set a wake and sleep schedule for every day of the week, including weekends. Your body temperature drops during sleep, so keep your thermostat at a cool, but comfortable, temperature between 60 and 70 degrees; avoid afternoon naps; try not to watch TV or do work in bed. Your brain needs time to unwind; if you typically exercise in the afternoon or evening, try to fit in your workout earlier in the day.

NAKED Tip

While there are no specific guidelines for how much relaxation a person should incorporate into their lifestyle, making time to unwind and enjoy life is an important part of maintaining good health. Deep relaxation, like meditation, when practiced regularly not only relieves stress and anxiety but is shown to improve mood. Deep relaxation has many other potential benefits as well—it can decrease blood pressure, relieve pain and improve your immune and cardiovascular systems.

Mind/Spirit Tip: Have Fun

When we hear the words "*spiritual wellbeing*," we tend to think of something mystical, even profound. It's neither, really. In fact, one of the most important aspects of our wellbeing is having fun.

When I rode my bicycle around my parents' driveway as a child, I didn't think of it as *exercise*, even though I was giving my heart a good workout. It was fun. Riding a bike is just a part of being a kid. For many of us, something changed along the path to adulthood. The idea of physical play became something you did with your children and not for yourself, if you did it at all. Whatever our activity of choice was—as kids—riding a bike, playing a sport, running around the schoolyard—it gradually became a chore. No one probably dragged you outdoors kicking and screaming to get you to ride your bike as a child. Now, when we need to jog, exercise or go to the gym, our first thought is often "Do I have to?"

So, how do we make the chore fun again?

For me, fun begins with a competitive challenge. Put me in a competition and it's game on. Think of the television show *The Biggest Loser*. That's my wheelhouse, and I'm not alone. We see competition everywhere in society. Just think about the massive popularity of game shows, elections and sporting events. Even the economy draws out a competitive spirit among business owners large and small. Some scholars believe competitiveness is a biological trait that co-evolved with our basic need for survival.

Knowing this trait lies inside each of us, take advantage of it! Even if that means competing with yourself, try setting a goal for your fitness plan every day, then pushing yourself to exceed your goals the next day. Anyone can do that much. Got high blood pressure? Take your reading one day at your local drug store, then see if you can lower it by your next visit.

If you can make physical activity fun again, you've killed two birds with one stone. Getting exercise won't feel like a chore but rather something you can look forward to. Playing video games, watching television, and playing card games with your friends can all be fun too, but these activities do nothing to nourish your body. When you exercise for fun, your body and spirit reap the benefits simultaneously. Now you're saving time too.

Science tells us the same chemicals (endorphins) released into our brain during distance running mimic the sense of euphoria felt by people who use opiates—codeine, OxyContin, Vicodin and the like. Some people are more prone to addiction than others, and the endorphin rush that comes with running has been known to turn cocaine and methamphetamine addicts into natural ultra-marathoners. But remember: baby steps. You might not feel the endorphins flowing if you can only walk around your block a couple times. Exercise-induced endorphin release is a goal you'll have to work toward. Even then, the more you exercise, the harder you'll have to work to feel an endorphin rush. Imagine that. Not only do our brains naturally reward us with pleasure for exercise, they push us to work harder too!

The science of fun is fascinating, but there's no need to complicate things. If the old saying is true about riding a bike, you can hop on one today no matter how long it's been since your last ride and enjoy a spin around your block. Give it a try, just for fun.

Day Fifteen

"Keeping busy and making optimism a way of life can restore your faith in yourself."

—Lucille Ball

This is the start of your third week on my program. You are well on your way to being in the best shape of your life.

Look at yourself in the mirror. Are you happy with the results so far? If so, that should be enough to push you to continue to reach your goals. If not, perhaps it's a sign you're not pushing yourself hard enough. Kick any obstacles in the butt, stay focused and look for small bits of motivation anywhere you can find it.

Rock your cardio and abs circuit today. Don't forget to stretch before and after your workout.

NAKED Tip

Need extra motivation today? Find a reason to get on that treadmill or pound the pavement or whatever you do to get that heart rate pumping. You're almost destined to fail without any motivation. Give yourself a fighting chance at sticking to your cardio regimen by thinking about *why* you want to get and stay active. It can be a broad reason like a desire to lose weight (though, a specific number should be the goal), or it can be a short-term goal like conditioning yourself for a race.

NAKED Tip

Another great motivator is to share your cardio success on social media. Just like having a training buddy, it helps you stay active and holds you accountable for your own success. I post a lot of pictures of my workouts and I take a lot of selfies. Quite frankly, this is the best body I've ever had in my life and I want to show it off. It's also a great way to receive compliments and words of encouragement from others, which in turn makes you want to work that much harder.

NAKED Tip

You're going to get from your cardio workouts only what you put into them. If you want great results, you have to put in a great effort. There are many ways to raise the intensity level of your workouts. The key is that you challenge yourself each and every session. You can run faster or longer, increase resistance, decrease the length of rest intervals, or push yourself a little harder in any other way you choose. Regardless, don't fall into the trap of simply going through the motions or clocking a certain amount of time. If your cardio workout feels easy, then you're not challenging yourself.

Mind/Spirit Tip: Embrace Change

As you've already discovered, the 30-day plan outlined here requires you to change your lifestyle. It's impossible to continue in the same pattern of behavior and feel better naked. Change isn't optional.

For most of us, change isn't desirable. It can be a very disruptive force. Some of us loathe change a little more than others. We're all creatures of habit to a degree, and for good reason: habits make life more convenient, our daily existence more comfortable. But being inflexible has drastic consequences for our minds and bodies.

In November 2004, the tech firm IBM hosted a Global Innovation Outlook conference. The company's top executives invited a team of experts from different disciplines and different countries to propose big solutions to big problems. One was health care. A renowned physician told the IBM audience "a relatively small percentage of the population consumes the vast majority of the health care budget for diseases that are very well-known and by and large behavioral." The solution? Well, there was none! The phenomenon hadn't changed in 50 years, because people persisted in their bad habits—smoking, drinking, poor diet, not enough exercise—even though they knew it was bad for them.

Using the example of coronary bypass surgery, an expensive and traumatic medical procedure related to heart disease, another doctor held up a startling statistic: two years after the bypass procedure, 90 percent of patients had not changed their lifestyles.

The lesson here isn't just that change can benefit us in the long run in powerful ways, to the point of saving our lives (though that's true, too). It's that your very nature *will* offer resistance to any drastic changes in your diet, exercise, or outlook on life. You'll have to fight for this.

Maybe no book better illustrates this concept than *Who Moved My Cheese?* by Spencer Johnson. When I owned a health club, it was required reading for all my employees. The book is about mice and men and a profound lesson, though it has nothing in common with the John Steinbeck classic. *Who Moved My Cheese?* focuses on change and how the four characters grapple with it. (The subject of the book isn't actually cheese; it's just a metaphor.)

You can probably read the book in an hour, though I'm not giving anything away by saying it teaches the correct way to grapple with change. The book follows the protagonist's journey through a literal maze. Along the way, he writes a series of messages on the walls that serve as powerful advice for the maze of life: "Change Happens," "Anticipate Change," "Monitor Change," "Adapt to Change Quickly," "Enjoy Change!" and "Be Ready To Change Quickly And Enjoy It Again and Again." Write those things down if you have to and commit them to memory. Your mind and spirit will be better for it.

Driving the same car, performing the same job or living in the same house might be a source of comfort, but what if your car is on the verge of breaking down, your job is killing you inside or your house is falling apart? These things happen—*life* happens—which is why being flexible is a fantastic habit to develop. Sometimes my gym employees would respond to a change in their daily tasks with a complaint: "You said we were going to do *this* today!"

"Well, guess what?" I would say. "It changed!"

Sometimes change is not an option. A new spouse, new baby, new job, new city or new house forces us to adapt to something disruptive. There will be big and small changes whether we like it or not. Sure, we can resist and complain, or we can accept the fact that the only constant in life *is* change. We can rely on death and taxes; nothing else will remain the same.

By changing your diet and exercise habits now, you aren't merely improving your health. You're embracing change, one of life's most difficult and most important skills to master.

Day Sixteen

"Resistance training is the only type of exercise that can slow, and even reverse, declines in muscle mass, bone density and strength that were once considered inevitable results of aging."
—Harvard Health Letter

Strength training is the closest thing we have to the Fountain of Youth. It is important in preventing the muscle loss that normally accompanies the aging process. A common misconception I used to always hear is that it's normal to stop being active when you reach a certain age. This couldn't be further from the truth. There is absolutely no reason why all of us can't be physically, mentally, socially, and sexually active, living a healthy vibrant life no matter our age.

Today, as you follow the same upper body weight training workout that you did on Day Two and Day Nine, focusing on your shoulders, back and arms, imagine you are taking a dip in the Fountain of Youth. Work hard and enjoy it!

Remember to change things up a bit by using a variation of upper body exercises found in Chapter Four. Drink plenty of fluids throughout this workout, and make sure you drink after as well.

Get your upper body ready for the workout with the **shoulder and arm warm-up**, and be sure to follow the proper form so you are getting the most out of your workout.

Circuit 1 (shoulder blast) standing or seated
Dumbbell (DB) front raise, 12—15 reps
Side lateral seated DB raises, 12—15 reps

Seated DB presses, 12—15 reps
DB upright rows, 12—15 reps
Repeat circuit three to five times
Rest period 30—45 seconds

Circuit 2 (back and arms)
Tricep high lateral rope pull-downs,12—15 reps
Speed rows using band in squatting position, 30—45 seconds
Tricep push-downs on cable machine, 15—20 reps
Standing bicep DB curls, 12—15 reps
Repeat circuit three to five times
Rest period 30—45 seconds

Circuit 3
One arm DB row on flat bench, 12—15 reps
Tricep kickbacks using DB, 15—20 reps
Seated concentration DB, curls 15—20 each arm
Repeat three to five times
Rest period 30—45 seconds

Circuit 4
Seated cable rows (machine), 12—15 reps
Standing tricep push-downs using tubing or bands, 12—15 reps
Standing bicep curls, 12—15 reps
Repeat three to five times
Rest period 30—45 seconds

At the end of your upper body workout, proceed to the abdominal circuit.

NAKED Tip

For women over 40, muscle mass can drop as much as ten percent, torpedoing your metabolism and boosting the odds of weight gain, which can double the risks of diabetes, heart disease, high blood pressure and stroke. Strength-training sessions help to rebuild muscle mass and benefit your bones, keeping them strong.

NAKED Tip

Bone density peaks by age 30, but through strength training, you can increase bone density and help prevent osteoporosis. Strength-training exercise increases your bone density by encouraging the release of growth hormone in your body, and it promotes new bone cell growth. Becoming stronger through exercise also protects your bones by helping you prevent falls which more commonly occur as you age.

NAKED Tip

Without stretching, our muscles tend to contract and tense up. Engaging in regular stretching sessions before and after working out helps elderly women decrease their likelihood of falling and remain flexible well into their later years.

Meal 1 (pre-workout)

Protein smoothie

1 scoop of protein powder shaken with 8 oz. of water.

NAKED Tip:

For those who prefer to have a protein shake with almond milk, it's naturally lactose free and free of cholesterol and saturated fat.

Meal 2 (post-workout)

¼ cup cream of rice cereal mixed in 1 cup of water

Boil the rice/water mixture in the microwave for about 3 minutes.

1 tsp of cinnamon sprinkled and/or a pinch of sea salt

NAKED Tip

Don't forget to always eat a breakfast and preferably one with a protein. Skipping breakfast, or even just having fruit, will not give you the energy you need to start your day.

Meal 3 (lunch salad with a protein)

1½ cup mixed greens, spinach, baby spinach, baby kale, or a mix of both

6—8 oz. lean meat

¼ cup of slivered almonds

1 tbsp. of dressing

NAKED Tip

Add ½ to 1 cup of garbanzo beans (chickpeas) to any salad. These are an excellent source of proteins, fiber and minerals.

Meal 4 (snack)

1 rice cake with 1 tbsp. raw peanut butter or raw almond butter spread on top.

NAKED Tip

Alternate snacks include: ¼ cup of raw or roasted almonds (no salt!), ¼ cup of walnuts, ¼ cup of berries or 1 apple.

Meal 5 (dinner)

6—8 oz. of salmon, cod or tilapia

Small side salad (e.g. 1 cup or less of spinach or kale) with chopped tomatoes and dressing

NAKED Tip

A great vegetable to add to your meal is artichoke hearts. Artichokes are a superfood, filled with antioxidants and fiber. You can buy them already prepared, heat them up in a microwave and serve alongside your fish; sprinkle with a little lemon or oil and vinegar.

Meal 6 (optional, can replace another meal or be a snack)

¼ cup of nuts

½ cup of berries

or

1 cup of popcorn, air popped and no butter, okay to season with a tbsp. herbs or spices

½ cup of berries

or

1 rice cake with 1 tbsp. of raw peanut butter or almond butter

¼ cup of berries

Mind/Spirit Tip: Relax

In the last chapter, I stressed the importance of being flexible and anticipating your mind's natural resistance to change. You also have to prepare your spirit for change. I've found the best way to do that is to look forward to the change and to make sure you have access to the relaxation tools and techniques that consistently work for you.

When you're changing your dietary habits, and working harder than you ever have to improve your body, be prepared for moments where you need to tell yourself to relax. If you don't tell yourself, don't be surprised if someone else tells you first! Have you ever been around someone who's having a bad day and they take it out on you? It's not fun.

Maybe you're a naturally relaxed person. If so, good for you. These days, it seems a lot of people don't know how to relax. The more items on your to-do list, the harder it becomes. Say you go on a vacation for a week. Many of us fret about leaving our lives behind: "If I'm away for that long, all this stuff won't get done!" So you're fried by the time getaway day comes because you've put in triple-time just to get there. Your first day away from home might be nauseating. It's supposed to be a time to relax, but you can't even calm down. Maybe you're fidgeting by the poolside. By the time you're not worried about checking emails and a sense of relaxation begins to sink in, your vacation is halfway over!

That's just one example, but it illustrates why we can't simply wait for an extended vacation to satisfy our need to relax. The next time your to-do list is spiraling out of control, set aside an hour of quiet time. Drinking a cup of coffee and reading a newspaper counts. Maybe close yourself off in a room, pretend you're sitting on a beach and feel the sand between your toes. A simple visualization exercise like that can go a long way.

Exercise, and its endorphin release, have been part of my wellbeing for years. So has meditation, which for me means escaping the hustle and bustle of life with a quiet moment of solitude. Many of my friends relax just by listening to music, doing yoga, watching TV, playing video games, getting a massage or stretching. It's important that you have *some* reliable tool at your disposal for those moments when you need to relax. Make sure you have ample time and access to these tools during any period of intense diet and exercise.

I also find comfort in reading (though when it's time to relax, I avoid thriller novels). Besides relaxing us, a good book comes with many positive side effects. Reading literary fiction has been shown to improve our skills in reading others' emotions. Any book has the capacity to improve your attention span, vocabulary, spatial awareness and ability to communicate.

If you enjoy drawing, doodling, painting or making any kind of art, these can be a great respite from chaos. The production of visual art has been shown to improve interaction between different parts of our brain. Research tells us artists are better observers and exhibit better memory than non-artists. Do you play an instrument? Playing music—not just listening—has been described as a "full body brain workout."

Whatever your preferred relaxation technique, be self-aware. Know when it's time to hit Pause on life. Your mind and spirit will be recharged when it's time to power up again.

Day Seventeen

"It always seems impossible until it's done."
—Nelson Mandela

Ready to get your cardio on?

Cardio exercise is not only great for weight loss, it also provides overall health benefits to the heart, lungs and circulation. While you're out there burning calories today think of all the great things you are doing for your body. That should be motivation enough!

Feeling great at the end of your workout? Push yourself to add on the extra core-training exercises recommended by my trainer. Core training is a fundamental part of fitness training and too often overlooked when working out. Core training improves overall performance and posture, alleviates lower back pain and tones and flattens the tummy.

Do your abs workout and really feel the burn.

NAKED Tip

If you're looking for another great outdoor cardio workout, put rollerblading at the top of your list. It will challenge your cardio fitness level while enhancing your lower-body strength. To help maximize results, try moving as low into the squat position as you can. The lower you go, the more you'll work out the glutes and quads, really adding to the overall benefits of the exercise.

NAKED Tip

If you don't feel motivated to get your heart rate pumping after work, pack a gym bag before you head out in the morning and bring it with you. This will prevent you from having to make a trip home where you can get lost in a sea of to-dos, and it also reinforces your after-work plans throughout the day as you glance at it sitting beside your desk.

<u>NAKED Tip</u>

Looking for a cardio exercise you can do right at home? Turn up the music and dance. This calorie-burning exercise is a fun way to break a sweat, and it keeps both the body and mind active, vital for people of every age.

Meal 1 (pre-workout)

Protein smoothie

1 scoop of protein powder shaken with 8 oz. of water.

<u>NAKED Tip</u>

Blueberries are a high fibrous fruit. If you wish to add fruit to your smoothie, blend in ½ cup of blueberries. This flavor profile may work with some protein powders and not others, so you will need to experiment.

Meal 2 (post-workout)

2 whole eggs, 1 egg white (cage free), 1 oz. baby spinach, 1 tsp coconut oil to make omelet; ⅛ tsp sea salt

<u>NAKED Tip</u>

When using olive oil, make sure it's extra virgin and cold pressed. Why? Because in extra virgin olive oil, the important antioxidants and anti-inflammatories have not been pressed out. It also tastes less acidic.

Meal 3 (lunch salad with a protein)

6—8 oz. grilled or sautéed shrimp

1 or 1 ½ cups mixed greens, spinach or kale

1 chopped tomato

Balsamic vinaigrette or olive oil and white vinegar mixture

Black pepper and sea salt to taste

<u>NAKED Tip</u>

The National Institute of Health (NIH) developed the Oxygen Radical Absorbance Capacity (ORAC) score to measure the antioxidant activity in a variety of fruits, vegetables and spices. At the top is ground cinnamon. At just one tablespoon, ground cinnamon can increase antioxidant levels in the blood higher than all the others listed. In the order listed after cinnamon are: red beans, blueberries, red kidney beans, pinto beans, cranberries, artichoke hearts, blackberries, prunes, raspberries, strawberries, red delicious apples, granny smith apples, pecans, sweet cherries, black plums, russet potatoes, black beans, plums and gala apples.

Meal 4 (snack)

2 celery stalks with raw peanut butter or raw almond butter

or

¼ cup almonds

or

1 avocado

or

1 apple

or

½ cup mixed berries

<u>NAKED Tip</u>

Oils you should avoid include canola oil, safflower oil, corn oil, sunflower oil and pure vegetable oil.

Meal 5 (dinner)

6—8 oz. lean turkey

1 cup of boiled broccoli, Brussels sprouts or cauliflower

<u>NAKED Tip</u>

A great salad a friend shared with me includes arugula with sliced pears and chopped walnuts. Use any simple vinaigrette dressing that isn't sweet because the pears have that covered.

Meal 6 (optional, can replace another meal or be a snack)

¼ cup of nuts

½ cup of berries

or
1 cup of popcorn, no butter, okay to season with a tbsp. herbs or spices
½ cup of berries
or
1 rice cake with 1 tbsp. of raw peanut butter or almond butter
¼ cup of berries

NAKED Tip

Pumpkin seeds are also high in fiber. A half cup of pumpkin seeds is a great snack, and you can bake them with a little extra virgin olive oil for an even tastier treat.

Mind/Spirit Tip: Volunteer

In 2006, a team of international researchers studied charitable donation behavior. What made the study unique was that the researchers weren't sociologists but neuroscientists. They weren't interested in who was giving money, or time, or talents, or who was receiving these things. They were interested in how the givers felt. Maybe you guessed the conclusion: the givers felt pretty good.

It gets better. Brain-imaging studies showed the "pleasure centers" in our brains—the parts of the brain that are active when we experience temporal pleasures like dessert, money and sex—are equally active when we observe someone giving money to charity as when we receive money ourselves. We're wired to volunteer like we're wired to procreate. Imagine that!

The first time I remember donating money, I was the charity case. I was a young girl, moving in and out of children's hospitals in Nebraska with rheumatic fever. The doctors and nurses were so nice to me. I can still remember turning to my mom as we left a hospital and asking if we could leave them some money.

Little did I know then that fundraising would become one of my missions as an adult. My ultimate reward is helping those in need. One of the more fun challenges for me now is finding creative ways to give. I once converted a room in my house—my closet—into a hub for charity events. I've climbed mountains, hosted fashion shows and thrown parties. Over time, I've found there are as many ways to raise money as there are people in need.

Before I did my charity climb up Mt. Kilimanjaro, I spent a week helping drill water wells in Malawi. Those are both unusual examples. The local homeless shelter, for example, doesn't need volunteers to climb a mountain. Giving to charity doesn't need to be creative, or complicated or even involve money or strenuous physical activity (though why not benefit your body, mind and someone in need at the same time?). Every charity organization in the world needs volunteers to do something. Many 501(c)(3) nonprofits accept cars, land or property as tax-deductible donations. A simple Internet search and a phone call is all it takes to find out who needs help and what you can do to assist. Just jump in, ask to tag along on a project and don't be afraid!

Remember, whether you're giving your time, your energy or your money, personal gain isn't the point. The point is always to help someone in need. If you're looking for glory, look elsewhere. Sometimes a flashy charity event is designed to bring recognition to the host. When going big, do it to attract big donors.

Fundraising and volunteering are seldom easy. The greater the reward, the harder it will be. To this day, it still isn't easy for me to persevere through the challenges of each fundraising project. A simple rule I live by helps me to push through: only give to something that evokes your passion. With enough passion for the cause or the people you're serving, it's possible to dig deep and overcome any obstacle.

I receive thousands of requests every month from people asking me for time or money. If the request doesn't tug at my heart or involve children—that's my passion—I don't take on the project. It's that simple.

For anyone with an urge to give, that's the starting point: find out what you're passionate about. We all have time and talents we can donate. Even fundraising doesn't require a large bank account—just enough time, energy, passion and persuasiveness to inspire others to give. It's one of the most rewarding things that absolutely anyone can do.

Day Eighteen

"Many of life's failures are people who did not realize how close they were to success when they gave up."
—Thomas A. Edison

Many people yearn for long, lean legs that fetch envious glances, but not all of us were born with it! If you're like me, you love to show off your legs, but you've got to work for it. Having strong leg muscles not only looks great in sexy skirts, shorts and dresses, it also helps with balance, mobility and a healthy back.

Today you're well on your way to sexy legs with the lower-body workout focusing on the legs and glutes. You will remember this workout from Day Four and Day Eleven. Be sure to begin with the hamstring glute stretch to get your muscles warmed up and ready to go.

Remember that variety is key, so swap out or add in any of the exercises for the legs and glutes from the list of exercises in Chapter Four. Drink plenty of water, and don't forget to complete your workout with the abdominal circuit.

Lower body circuit (45 to 60 minutes)

Five-minute warm-up
Leg extensions, 15—20 reps, four sets

Circuit 1

Smith machine squats, 15—20 reps
Walking lunges, 50—75 yards
Seated or kneeling leg curls machine, 15—20 reps
Repeat three to four sets
Rest period 30—45 seconds

Circuit 2

Seated leg press (machine), 15—20 reps
Standing body weight squats, 30—40 reps
Anterior reach lunge 12—15 each leg
Repeat four to five times
Rest period 30—45 seconds

Circuit 3

Jump squats 30 seconds
Alternating jumping lunges 30 seconds
Repeat three to four times
Rest period 30—45 seconds

Circuit 4

Lying glute bridge off stability ball, legs straight 15—20 reps
Lying glute bridge with knees bent, feet flat resistance ball, pushing hips up as high as you can 15—20 reps
Lying leg curls on stability ball 15—20 reps
Repeat three to four times
Rest period 30—45 seconds

<u>NAKED Tip</u>

Don't skip your leg day. Having strong legs not only helps improve cardio performance but helps us manage our overall body weight. The leg muscles are some of the biggest muscles in the body, so if we make them bigger and stronger, our body fat will be easier to manage. More muscle burns more fuel, and body fat will decrease with that. By training our legs, our bodies burn through a lot more fuel and release a lot more hormones that help us maintain body composition a lot easier.

<u>NAKED Tip</u>

If you try a new exercise or exercise at a higher level of intensity, your muscles may be sore in the days after your workout. This is because the increased intensity puts a strain on the muscles you used, causing very small tears in the muscle fibers. As the muscles heal, they grow back stronger and are better able to work at a higher level of intensity. Here some things you can do to help relieve muscle soreness.

- Gentle stretching
- Muscle massage
- Ice to help reduce inflammation
- Heat to help stimulate blood flow to the muscle
- Rest
- Over-the-counter pain medicine, such as a nonsteroidal anti-inflammatory drug (NSAID)

NAKED Tip

If you have an injury, you'll probably want to do whatever you can to make sure you don't miss a workout, but this is not always the best idea. If you continue training, or return to training too soon, you can increase your chance of developing a chronic injury that may never fully go away.

On the other hand, if you take too much time off, you will lose much of what you worked so hard to build. If you're like me, you won't want to miss any time at all because of an injury, so here are a few tips that will help you effectively train with an injury so you won't miss significant time away from the gym.

- Avoid inflammation-promoting foods such as fried foods, processed white flour, eggplant, tomatoes and cayenne, and eat more foods that are high in Omega-3 fatty acids.
- Be sure to drink plenty of juices made from fresh, organic, raw veggies, because raw veggies are high in important enzymes and vitamins that can speed up the healing process.
- Know when to tough it out. Most of the time, it is a good idea to just stop and heal up before training again.
- Train with lighter weights and higher reps.

Meal 1 (pre-workout)

Protein smoothie

1 scoop of protein powder shaken with 8 oz. of water.

NAKED Tip

Black tea is a great because it is high in antioxidants and helps reduce the risk of stroke. Some research shows that women who drink black tea regularly reduce their risk of ovarian cancer.

Meal 2 (post-workout)

Awesome omelet
1 large egg
4 egg whites
½ tsp. sea salt
1 tbsp. freshly chopped cilantro
¼ cup chopped onion
¼ cup black beans
¼ cup tomatoes

NAKED Tip

Onions not only add great flavor to many meals, they also lower blood glucose levels and contribute to lowering the risk in heart disease due to their lower LDL cholesterol and triglyceride levels.

Meal 3 (lunch salad with a protein)

1 can of white tuna in water
1 cup mix of chopped broccoli, cauliflower, red onion and celery
Mix ¼ cup of olive oil with 3 tablespoons lemon juice, 2 tablespoons soy sauce, 1 tsp mustard.

NAKED Tip

Whatever you eat during the NAKED Program, avoid white potatoes. White potatoes are high in GI rating, which means they convert to glucose rapidly.

Meal 4 (snack)

2 celery stalks with raw peanut butter or raw almond butter

NAKED Tip

The top food sources of iron include: egg yolks, red meat, dark leafy greens, artichokes, calf's liver, oysters, clams, scallops, turkey, beans, lentils, chickpeas, soybeans, dried prunes, raisins apricots and dates.

Meal 5 (dinner)

6—8 oz. flank steak, cooked to taste
1½ cup baby kale
1 cup chopped tomatoes
Salt and pepper to taste

NAKED Tip

Eating more regularly can literally help avoid depression. Why? Because when your blood sugar is low, among the side effects, which include fatigue and irritability, comes depression.

Meal 6 (optional, can replace another meal or be a snack)

¼ cup of nuts

½ cup of berries

or

1 cup of popcorn, no butter, okay to season with a tbsp. herbs or spices

½ cup of berries

or

1 rice cake with 1 tbsp. of raw peanut butter or almond butter

¼ cup of berries

NAKED Tip

The top complex carbohydrates include: nuts, raisins, vegetables, fruits, legumes, barley, brown and wild rice, sweet potatoes, winter squash and oats.

Mind/Spirit Tip: Find Your Motivation in Everything

Before I married my husband, I dated a man with a hidden talent. He had no idea at the time, but he was a fantastic motivational speaker. I didn't discover the talent until the day we broke up. I was trying to win a bodybuilding competition, the 1999 U.S. Open. As he turned and walked away from me for good, the last thing he said was that I'd never win the competition. Those were exactly the words I needed to hear to get my butt in gear. Four months later, I won.

Knowing someone else doesn't believe in you is precisely what it takes to accomplish a goal sometimes. If anyone's ever told you that you can't lose weight, stick with a program for 30 days or look good naked, great! Never forget the feeling of being doubted. Hold onto it—it might just be your best friend.

I discovered this surprising truth at an early age. When I was a little girl, a doctor diagnosed me with a heart murmur and said I was going to be a sickly child. I would never be normal, I would have to spend my days indoors and I couldn't be a mother because childbirth would be too taxing on my heart. Those words definitely got my heart racing. I was determined to prove the doctor wrong—and I did.

Some days, we want to be inspired. Sunday-morning sermons in church usually fill me with enough inspiration to last a week. Other times reading a book, listening to a song or watching a movie will do just fine. Then there are those unsettling times when inspiration slaps us right in the face so hard we don't realize what hit us. Maybe it's an angry ex, a discouraging doctor's report or even tragedy.

At my younger brother's funeral, I stood and listened as friends and colleagues from the air force remembered all my brother accomplished in his short life. He had earned more medals in his 23 years than I'd touched in my 28. I never expected a medal for being a great mom, but I couldn't help but think: *I'm his older sister and I haven't done half of these things in my life. What else do I want to be remembered for?* That melancholy moment served as motivation, too.

Since that day, I've set out to do some memorable things. I climbed Mt. Kilimanjaro and dug water wells in Africa, only to be inspired by the villagers' humble joy. I've raised thousands of dollars for non-profits in dire need. These endeavors have allowed me to give motivational speeches, which is always an honor.

You don't need to be standing at a pulpit or climbing a mountain to inspire another person. A casual conversation or a word of encouragement can go a long way. I'm often amazed by how inspiration can come from anyone at anytime. Whether I'm talking to a group of people or just one person low on inspiration, I like to remind them that being at the lowest point in life allows us to appreciate the highest peaks that much more.

After I won the U.S. Open of bodybuilding, my then ex-boyfriend called to congratulate me. I'll never forget what he told me: "I knew you would win!" He'll never know how much more the sincere insult meant than the phony compliment.

Day Nineteen

"Keep your face always toward the sunshine, and shadows will fall behind you."
—Walt Whitman

Today is your last cardio day of the week, so make it count. For a fun workout get on the elliptical machine at the gym. It raises your heart rate even more than the treadmill.

Here are some ideas for a challenging elliptical routine:

- Do five-minute intervals increasing resistance each time.
- Start and stay with a steady pace and increase the machine's incline/decline setting.
- Move at base-pace for two minutes, then double the speed for two minutes (keeping incline steady) and recover for one minute. Repeat this pattern as many times as desired.

Complete your abdominal circuit, and remember to hydrate often.

NAKED Tip

Whether you're a serious athlete or a recreational exerciser, it's important to make sure you get the right amount of water before, during, and after exercise. If you're not properly hydrated, your body can't perform at its highest level. The American Council on Exercise has suggested the following basic guidelines for drinking water before, during and after exercise:

- Drink 17—20 ounces of water two to three hours before you start exercising
- Drink eight ounces of water 20—30 minutes before you start exercising or during your warm-up
- Drink 7—10 ounces of water every 10—20 minutes during exercise
- Drink eight ounces of water no more than 30 minutes after you exercise

NAKED Tip

To avoid injuring yourself during exercise, don't try to do too much too soon. Start with an activity that is fairly easy for you, such as walking or light jogging. Slowly increase the amount of time and the intensity of the activity. Pay attention to your body. Stop exercising if you feel very out of breath, dizzy, faint, or nauseous, or if you feel pain.

NAKED Tip

Regular physical activity is good for your brain. Studies have shown that people who do simple exercises on a regular basis are better able to make decisions than people who aren't physically active.

Meal 1 (pre-workout)

Protein smoothie

1 scoop of protein powder shaken with 8 oz. of water.

NAKED Tip

Honey is a great sweetener because it contains natural anti-inflammatory properties and provides support to your arteries. Honey naturally contains caffeic acid, known to help prevent the formation of precancerous tissue.

Meal 2 (post-workout)

2 eggs, 1 egg white (cage-free) for scrambled eggs or omelet with:

¼ cup chopped red onion

½ chopped green pepper

⅓ cup spinach

NAKED Tip

Beware of agave syrup. It has been well marketed as a health food but is in fact very highly processed, so much so that it is a high-fructose syrup just like corn syrup and has the same harmful effects on your blood sugar.

Meal 3 (lunch salad with a protein)

6—8 oz. grilled skinless chicken breast

1½ cup mixed greens, spinach, baby spinach, baby kale, or a mix of both

¼ cup of slivered almonds

1 tbsp. of dressing

NAKED Tip

Diet sodas literally cause weight gain. They confuse your body's ability to know when it is full by bypassing the leptin response—leptin is a protein that tells your body when it is full—and the outcome is that you eat more!

Meal 4 (snack)

1—2 cups of kale to make crispy kale chips

Spread raw kale leaves on a cookie sheet sprayed with olive oil

Drizzle 1 tablespoon of olive oil over the kale leaves and top with pinch of sea salt

Cook at 375 degrees until crispy

NAKED Tip

Top tips for conquering cravings: eat protein, drink a lot of water, choose nuts as a snack, choose raw veggies as a snack and do not skip meals.

Meal 5 (dinner)

6—8 oz. grilled skinless chicken breasts, sliced into strips

1—2 cups mixed greens

¼ red onion, sliced in long, thin slices

½ cup black beans

1 tablespoon dressing.

NAKED Tip

Sugar will literally wreak havoc on the body. Among the many terrible outcomes, please consider these: it adds to your weight and girth, triggers inflammation, leads to diabetes, cardiovascular disease and cancer, can ruin your eyesight and can damage your arteries.

Meal 6 (optional, can replace another meal or be a snack)

¼ cup of nuts

½ cup of berries

or

1 cup of popcorn, no butter, okay to season with a tbsp. herbs or spices

½ cup of berries

or

1 rice cake with 1 tbsp. of raw peanut butter or almond butter

¼ cup of berries

NAKED Tip

The best way to continue getting healthy involves building a great support system. Whether that's your parents, spouse, other family members or friends, you need support to make this transition.

Mind/Spirit Tip: Think Positively

There's a popular preacher in Texas named Joel Osteen. By his own admission, the purpose of his Sunday sermons is not to emphasize the consequences of sin, but rather to "focus on the goodness of God" in order to "give people a boost for the week." Interestingly, Osteen doesn't take a salary from his church, which eventually grew from 5,000 to 50,000 attendees after he took over for his father in 1999.

Some have disagreed with Osteen's approach to theology, but that's beside the point. The point is to highlight the power of positive thought. It attracts people like moths to a flame. One reason Joel Osteen doesn't take a salary from his church is because he doesn't need to. His books, which include titles like *Become a Better You* and *Love YourLife* have sold enough copies around the world to make him a millionaire many times over. People thrive on being inspired, and being inspired comes from thinking positively. Have you ever attended a motivational speech? It's all positive talk and positive thinking. You feel so pumped, you'll walk away ready to light the world on fire.

The opposite is also true. I'm still waiting to meet the person who says, "I trace my success back to the day I threw a pity party for myself." When I'm around negative people, it brings my energy down to zero. They suck the energy right out of me, and I become one of them. I have to maintain my distance or ultimately walk away. From my experience, whether you think positively or negatively is entirely within your control. If you're a negative thinker, people simply won't be attracted to your spirit.

So what do I do when I'm in a bad mood? I smile, pull my big girl panties on and think, "Okay, let's go!" Think positively. It will get you everywhere in life. This is one area in which performance artists and scientists can both agree.

Emma Seppala, author of *The Happiness Track: How to Apply the Science of Happiness to Accelerate Your Success*, identified four concrete ways in which happiness brings out our best potential:

1. Positive emotions help you learn faster, think more creatively and resolve challenging situations. One study showed that people have an easier time solving a puzzle after watching a short comedy clip.
2. By helping you recuperate from negative emotions, positive emotions shorten the time you feel stressed, angry or depressed. Say you're stuck in bumper-to-bumper traffic but you just found out you're going to become a parent or a grandparent. That happiness can quickly relieve the tension created by your environment.
3. Positive emotions boost our inclination to connect with others in productive ways, while negative feelings like anxiety and depression leave us more self-centered. This has huge implications for the way we interact with our coworkers.
4. Positive emotions actually improve your physical wellbeing by increasing strength and cardiovascular health as well as coordination, sleep and immune function. Positive emotions are also associated with reduced inflammation.

Since your body will no doubt feel some pain during this 30-day program, let's focus on the last point. Further research shows optimists recover better from medical procedures such as coronary bypass surgery and live longer—both in general and when suffering from conditions such as cancer, heart disease and kidney failure.

So, what's a little exercise-induced pain? Tell yourself it'll be okay. There's an excellent chance you'll be right.

Day Twenty

"Never confuse a single defeat with a final defeat."
—F. Scott Fitzgerald

The last workout day of the week can be so inspiring. Knowing you're at the end of a grueling week of working out should lift your spirits and motivate you to perform at your highest level yet. Go get 'em!

We return to the upper-body series of strength training exercises targeting the chest, shoulders and back. You will recognize the strength-training circuit from Day Five and Day Thirteen.

Increase the amount of reps to failure, and then push yourself to do one more. But, don't compromise your form.

Do your **shoulder and arm warm-up**. Drink plenty of water, and don't forget to complete your workout with the abdominal circuit.

Circuit 1 (back)

Lat pull-downs, 3 sets of 15 reps
Seated rows, 3 sets of 15 reps
Assisted pull-ups, 3 sets of 15 reps
Repeat three to five times
Rest period 30—45 seconds

Circuit 2 (chest)

Standard push-ups 20 reps
Dumbbell presses, three sets of 15
Reverse push-ups on the resistance ball
Repeat three to five times
Rest period 30—45 seconds

Circuit 3 (shoulders)

Dumbbell (DB) front raises, 12—15 reps
Side lateral seated DB raises, 12—15 reps
Seated DB presses, 12—15 reps
DB upright rows, 12—15 reps
Repeat circuit three to five times
Rest period 30—45 seconds

NAKED Tip

If you don't have weights, look for items around your house that can act as a weight. Use a can of soup, a book or a full bottle of water. Keep your weights in the same room as your television and do a few exercises while you watch TV.

NAKED Tip

Unless an injury is serious, I always try to find a way to work around it. For example, if you have an elbow problem, you may want to try using alternative movements instead of normal movements. Try changing your grip on the weight, or see if alternative exercises for the same muscle group cause the same pain.

NAKED Tip

Don't skip your push-ups. They help to build strong pectoral (chest) muscles. Strong pec muscles not only enhance a woman's appearance in a bathing suit and in clothes, but are essential when it comes to posture, movement and power.

Meal 1 (pre-workout)

Protein smoothie
1 scoop of protein powder shaken with 8 oz. of water.

NAKED Tip:

Blueberry leaf extract (BLE) is a great supplement for helping drive down glucose levels and inflammation. You can buy BLE in capsule form to be taken before meals. It is also a good remedy for natural pain relief and eczema.

Meal 2 (post-workout)

¼ cup cream of rice cereal mixed in 1 cup of water

Boil the rice/water mixture in the microwave for about three minutes. If you use more water, the mixture is more watery like farina; less water and it's chunkier like a pudding.

1 tsp of cinnamon sprinkled on top

Pinch of sea salt

Meal 3 (lunch salad with a protein)

1½ cup mixed greens, spinach, baby spinach, baby kale, or a mix of both

6—8 oz. of lean meat

¼ cup of slivered almonds

1 tbsp. of dressing

NAKED Tip

Fish oil is loaded with DHA (docosahexaenoic acid), which has a profound effect on your health. It slows the liver's production of undesirable triglycerides, helps lower blood pressure and increase blood circulation and is effective at reducing inflammation.

Meal 4 (snack)

1 rice cake with 1 tbsp. raw peanut butter or raw almond butter spread on top

NAKED Tip

Labels are riddled with words to camouflage the presence of added sweeteners. These include: high-fructose corn syrup, maltose, maple syrup, corn sweetener, natural sweeteners, juice concentrate, lactose, dextrose, sucrose and molasses.

NAKED Tip

Fish naturally pairs nicely with spring greens and asparagus. Add minced shallots and grated lemon rind to add more flavor, along with a nice vinaigrette of extra-virgin olive oil.

Meal 5 (dinner)

6—8 oz. of salmon

Small side salad (e.g. 1 cup or less of spinach or kale) with chopped tomatoes and dressing

NAKED Tip

Many of us want a drink with dinner, and I don't mean soda, I mean alcohol. Here's the deal: alcohol prevents fat burning. It can slow the metabolism and puts your liver in overdrive trying to clear it from the bloodstream, which leaves the glucose to be converted to body fat instead of energy.

Meal 6 (optional, can replace another meal or be a snack)

¼ cup of nuts
½ cup of berries
or
1 cup of popcorn, air popped and no butter, okay to season with a tbsp. herbs or spices
½ cup of berries
or
1 rice cake with 1 tbsp. of raw peanut butter or almond butter
¼ cup of berries

NAKED Tip

A nice bubbly drink you can enjoy is sparkling water or seltzer with a wedge of lemon or lime.

Mind/Spirit Tip: Don't Complain

In the movie *Airplane!*, there's a scene in which two passengers are sitting next to each other. One is wearing a Japanese general's World War II uniform. The other man begins to unload all his life's problems as the general dutifully listens. The scene cuts away to a flashback; minutes later, we cut back to the airplane to see the general has committed suicide rather than listen to the other man drone on about his problems.

By now, you understand the power of positive thought. You can take an insult or a tragedy and turn it into a source of motivation. You know that fun isn't something you were supposed to leave behind in your childhood. Still, we all like to complain, and we can always find *something* to complain about. Some of us don't have to look for it at all—we simply do it out of habit.

Truth be told, I was the Japanese general on an airplane once, sitting next to someone who wanted to complain about all their problems in life. Maybe he found it therapeutic to unburden his conscience to a stranger, but look at the bigger picture: we never know what the person next to us is going through. Our ingrown toenail, painful though it may be, would be dwarfed by the next person's terminal cancer. When I was grieving the loss of my son and my brother, I didn't have the heart to share those details with every person who reflexively asked how I was doing. Saying "Horrible, thanks for asking!" does nothing to improve the other person's mood or to relieve my own anxiety.

The lesson: *Nothing is worth complaining about*. Nobody's life is perfect, but why moan? Unless you know someone very well, the question of "how are you today?" probably isn't an invitation to unload your life's problems. Chances are they don't *really* care about how you're doing today; they just don't know what else to say.

I didn't stab myself in the stomach that day on the airplane. I plugged my earbuds into my ears and pretended to listen to music. I decided I'd rather come across as rude than be dragged down by someone else's negative energy.

Maybe that sounds selfish, but consider this: body-language studies have touted the virtues of smiling for years. It's been proven that without practice, smiling muscles weaken and wither. Bitterness, sadness and anger reposition your muscles into a "downturned smile." Instead of smiling, a pouching at the corner of the mouth pulls your grin downward. Allan Pease, a body-language expert and author of *The Definitive Bookof Body Language*, has been quoted as saying that your face "becomes a permanent record of emotions throughout one's own life. There's the old expression 'After 40, your face is your fault,' but in fact it's even way before that."

Maybe you have a lot to complain about when you look in the mirror. If you've neglected your physical wellbeing for a long time, I'd be surprised if you didn't! Here's a strategy: try to visualize yourself standing in front of the mirror, naked, except this time you're happy with what you see. You have nothing to complain about. You probably aren't frowning. Your facial muscles are turning up, and you didn't miss out on the benefits of complaining instead. That's because there are none!

Will Bowen, author of *A Complaint Free World: How to Stop Complaining and Start Enjoying the Life You Always Wanted* suggests we need 21 consecutive days to turn a behavior into a habit. So he challenges readers to go 21 consecutive days without complaining. You might think a three-week period of intense diet and exercise is the worst time to take up such a challenge, but I'd argue it's the best time. If you can eradicate complaining from your life now, it will only be easier later on.

Even when you feel like complaining, next time don't complain—and you might not feel like complaining anymore!

Day Twenty-One

"Rest is vital to your weight loss, your health, and your ability to build muscle."
—TheFitTutor.com

Congratulations on completing week three of my NAKED Program! Celebrate your hard work and accomplishments thus far with a day of rest, which is important to recharge your mind and body.

A rest can actually rekindle your hunger for exercise and help prevent burnout, but if you're feeling antsy for some physical activity, take a stroll on the beach (if you live near one) or take a scenic bike ride through your neighborhood. You'll be glad you did.

NAKED Tip

Pilates is great workout for a rest day. It hits your core unlike any other workout. It helps reduce lower back pain, it's easy on the joints and it improves your flexibility and overall workout performance. However, Pilates classes are not cheap because of the high cost of Pilates instructor training, the extensive level of expertise that such training imparts and the overhead associated with providing and maintaining Pilates equipment. To make Pilates fit your budget, try at-home videos or online workouts.

NAKED Tip

Consider a reflexology treatment on rest day. Reflexology aims to reduce the effects of stress and tension in the body, thereby aiding recovery and muscle repair and helping to moderate fatigue and soreness. One of the results after a reflexology treatment is a deep feeling of relaxation and a release of stress and tension. Reflexology provides a similar response to a massage therapy; although the main difference is that the therapy is applied at a point distant to the injury or soreness. This makes it a more pleasant experience. After a reflexology treatment I often feel like I've just gotten a deep tissue massage even though only my feet were touched!

<u>NAKED Tip</u>

Sleep is a very important factor to consider with regard to muscle recovery. When you lift weights, your muscle fibers are breaking down and tearing. It is the repairing of those small tears that makes the muscle stronger, and sleep is essential in maintaining strong muscles. An added bonus of exercise: most people who exercise regularly fall asleep faster and sleep more soundly!

Mind/Spirit Tip: Check Your Envy at the Door

Envy is a devious emotion that afflicts us all. Whether it burns like an inferno or merely flickers in the background, the pilot light is always lit, ready to burst into flames at the mere thought of craving something that isn't ours. "If you desire glory, you may envy Napoleon," the philosopher Bertrand Russell once said, "but Napoleon envied Caesar, Caesar envied Alexander, and Alexander, I daresay, envied Hercules, who never existed."

Rather than wasting time wanting what someone else has, spare your mind and spirit the pain. Set attainable goals and work for them. My mother taught me at a very young age that someone else will always be smarter, prettier and more talented than I am. It's good to strive to be the best, or at least something more than what you are today. But if you fall short, you can at least save yourself a lot of time by accepting your shortcomings and being happy for those who have more.

Why, then, can't we just "get over it?" For one thing, our brains are hard-wired for envy. A team of researchers at the National Institute of Radiological Sciences in Japan found that the region of our brain that processes envy is also involved in processing physical pain. In short, envy really hurts. Our brains are also wired for *schadenfreude*—taking pleasure when someone we envy experiences misfortune. The same team of researchers found that the *schadenfreude* region of our brain also lights up when we eat something delicious. Maybe the words to the theme song of *The Jeffersons* were really onto something: "I finally got a piece of the pie!"

Of course, George Jefferson operated a successful dry-cleaning business. He worked for his deluxe apartment in the sky. I could never understand the envy of those who aren't willing to work for the things they crave. Why waste time envying what others possess when you can work hard to obtain it? And yet, if you type a celebrity's name into Google—even if they're only a little famous—*net worth* is often one of the first suggested search terms that follows. Maybe you never had any desire to know that person's net worth, but it's clear what others are interested in finding out: how big is their pie?

Envy comes in many shapes and sizes. I know of moms who try to one-up their neighbors by throwing lavish birthday parties for their young children. Or what about the billionaire who bought two rare diamonds for his seven-year-old daughter at a reported cost of $77 million? By putting common sense ahead of their oversized egos, these people would save their time and money—and their young children probably wouldn't mind one bit!

Don't fool yourself. If you're human, you're prone to envy. It's an integral function of our brains. However, that's not an excuse to allow envy to evolve into hatred. We don't really hate the people who have the things we want. We just want a piece of the pie. So don't waste a second wallowing in your envy—go out and work for it!

Day Twenty-Two

"Never give in. Never give in. Never, never, never, never—in nothing, great or small, large or petty—never give in, except to convictions of honor and good sense. Never yield to force. Never yield to the apparently overwhelming might of the enemy."
—Winston S. Churchill

I've heard many times that is takes 21 days to build a habit. Welcome to Day 22! You're at the finish line—the last full week of my NAKED Program. But, you're not done yet! Push yourself harder this week than ever before and finish the program strong.

Today is cardio day. We've talked all throughout this book about how important it is to change things up to prevent boredom and really make the most of your workouts. Why not add a few jumping jacks to your cardio routine? Not only are jumping jacks an effective cardio workout, they also strengthen joints and improve oxygen levels in the body, which gives a boost to blood circulation.

You can find tons of jumping jack variations on the Internet, from standard to plank to twist and star, so make them a part of your cardio routine today.

Do your abs routine and try to get as close to your 20 reps as possible. Don't forget to hydrate!

NAKED Tip

Some people have a harder time making exercise a habit than others. Here are some ways to help those who need an extra push:

- Stick to a regular time every day.
- Sign a contract committing yourself to exercise.
- Put "exercise appointments" on your calendar.
- Keep a daily log or diary of your exercise activities.
- Check your progress. Can you walk a certain distance faster now? Are you at your target heart rate?
- Think about joining a health club or community center. The cost might give you an incentive to exercise on a regular basis.

NAKED Tip

Sometimes workouts get skipped because you're sick. Or because of travel and busy schedules. If you miss a day (or two or three), just get back at it as if nothing has happened, starting with the workout you skipped. If you miss much longer you'll have to decide whether you want to start the program over from scratch or ramp yourself back up to the place you were when you stopped. Either way, dig deep to find the motivation to reach your goals.

NAKED Tip

Here are some tried and true tips for workout success:

- Always carry a bottle of water with you wherever you go.
- Don't look at exercise as a burden or a chore. Think positive and get excited for your workouts.
- Focus on completing one exercise routine at a time. Otherwise, you're in danger of feeling overwhelmed.
- Avoid boredom by changing up your exercises.
- A new pair of sneakers or workout gear will help you stay motivated and inspired.

Meal 1 (pre-workout)

Protein smoothie

1 scoop of protein powder shaken with 8 oz. of water.

NAKED Tip:

Green tea has been shown to stabilize blood sugar and improve kidney, liver and pancreatic function. It helps alleviate arthritis, prevent viral infections and manage allergies. The list goes on, so don't be shy about enjoying a daily dose of hot green tea.

Meal 2 (post-workout)

¼ cup cream of rice cereal mixed in 1 cup of water

Boil the rice/water mixture in the microwave for about 3 minutes. If you use more water, the mixture is more watery like farina; less water and it's chunkier like a pudding. This is a personal preference, so discover which you prefer.

1 tsp of cinnamon sprinkled on top

Pinch of sea salt

NAKED Tip

Fruit juice can elevate blood sugar and make you feel hungry and crave sweets. The exceptions to this rule include tomato juice, blueberry juice or unsweetened pomegranate juice mixed with seltzer.

Meal 3 (lunch salad with a protein)

1½ cup mixed greens, spinach, baby spinach, baby kale, or a mix of both

6—8 oz. of lean meat

¼ cup of slivered almonds

1 tbsp. of dressing

NAKED Tip

Add some excitement to water by accessorizing with lemons, cucumbers, mint or limes. You can slice lemons, cucumbers and limes and let the slices soak in a tall glass of water for a while to infuse the water with the flavors. Do the same with some fresh mint leaves.

Meal 4 (snack)

1 rice cake with 1 tbsp. raw peanut butter or raw almond butter spread on top

NAKED Tip

Foods loaded with carbohydrates that you want to avoid include: pancakes, waffles, bagels, French toast, muffins, doughnuts, cupcakes, white bread, soda, pastries, white rice, French fries, hash browns, tortillas, and boxed cereals.

NAKED Tip

Cancer, arthritis, diabetes and obesity have been linked to inflammation. The top foods that cause inflammation include: sugar, pizza and cheese, cookies, doughnuts, crackers, mayonnaise and many salad dressings, breads, rolls, French fries, white rice, white potatoes, most pasta, dairy and wheat.

Meal 5 (dinner)

6—8 oz. of salmon

Small side salad (e.g. 1 cup or less of spinach or kale) with chopped tomatoes and dressing

NAKED Tip

Squeeze some lemon on your salmon to give it some flavor, or even sprinkle some seasonings on while it bakes.

Meal 6 (optional, can replace another meal or be a snack)

¼ cup of nuts

½ cup of berries

or

1 cup of popcorn, air popped and no butter, okay to season with a tbsp. herbs or spices

½ cup of berries

or

1 rice cake with 1 tbsp. of raw peanut butter or almond butter

¼ cup of berries

NAKED Tip

Try vegetarian refried beans as a snack. Mix with some chopped tomatoes and a bit of salsa.

Mind/Spirit Tip: Live in the moment

When I was single, I dated a man so busy preparing for the future that he wasn't living in the present. One night we were getting ready to go out to dinner and he said, "Let's see, if I spend $40 on dinner tonight, that's $40 not going into my retirement account." He was so hell-bent on his 401(k)s and IRAs that he couldn't enjoy going out for dinner. Talk about penny pinching! I can only hope his retirement accounts outlasted our relationship.

I've also met people who have the opposite problem: they dwell on the past. Whether it be past relationships or past accomplishments, successes or failures, their minds seem to be somewhere else. Sometimes their focus is on recapturing something they lost. Sometimes they can't get past a poor choice that's still weighing down their conscience. My advice: acknowledge it, then bury it. Move on and live in the moment.

I admit living in the moment is easier said than done. Tomorrow's plans are always pulling us away. Smartphones, tablets, laptops and TVs are addictive, tugging at your brain to divert your attention. And the past always seems happier than the present. Our brains are even wired to think so. Psychologist Art Markman explains why: "When we look back on events from our youth, we are likely to remember many things as being excellent, or awesome, or brilliant. We just forget how we decided on their excellence or brilliance. With a broader base of experience as an adult, it takes a lot for us to be truly awed. So we decide that things must have been better when we were younger."

I think when I lost my 19-year-old son in a car accident, and my 23-year-old brother to a heart attack, it dawned on me that I could be taken tomorrow too. With no promise of a new day, I better start enjoying my life. Knowing every moment could be your last when you go to bed, you tend to appreciate it more.

That doesn't mean don't plan for the future. When you set aside time to make a list, or to plan ahead, be in that moment. There's value in reflecting on the past too, and research offers a good reason to strive for some balance. In a paper published in the *Journal of Positive Psychology*, a team of researchers identified the difference between a happy life and a meaningful life: "...happiness is about the present, whereas meaning is about linking events across time, thus integrating past, present, and future. Meaning links experiences and events across time, whereas happiness is mostly in the moment and therefore largely independent of other moments. The more time people reported having devoted to thinking about the past and future, the more meaningful their lives were—and the less happy."

The takeaway: you can't spend all your time planning or reflecting, even though those activities will help add meaning to your life. Say you have an important business meeting in the coming days or an unresolved argument lingering from the night before. Maybe that's a good time to do the laundry. Dig deep into your brain. Get some heavy thinking out of the way while you fold the whites.

Then, focus on the present. You'll be happier. The people around you will appreciate the attention you're giving them, certainly more than your retirement plan ever will.

Remember, you'll never be younger than you are now, but you always can feel younger than you did yesterday.

Day Twenty-Three

"Real courage is when you know you're licked before you begin, but you begin anyway and see it through no matter what."
—Harper Lee, *To Kill a Mockingbird*

Today, as you work through your upper-body strength training routine, think of where you were when you started this circuit a few weeks ago. You probably couldn't have imagined getting to this point in the program. You're stronger today than you were just a few weeks ago, so keep going and continue to find the motivation to help you reach your goals.

Get your upper body ready for the workout with the **shoulder and arm warm-up**, and be sure to follow the proper form so you are getting the most out of your workout.

Circuit 1 (shoulder blast) standing or seated
Dumbbell (DB) front raise, 12—15 reps
Side lateral seated DB raises, 12—15 reps
Seated DB presses, 12—15 reps
DB upright rows, 12—15 reps
Repeat circuit three to five times
Rest period 30—45 seconds

Circuit 2 (back and arms)
Triceps high lateral rope pull-downs,12—15 reps
Speed rows using band in squatting position, 30—45 seconds
Triceps push-downs on cable machine, 15—20 reps
Standing bicep DB curls, 12—15 reps
Repeat circuit three to five times
Rest period 30—45 seconds

Circuit 3

One arm DB row on flat bench, 12—15 reps
Triceps kickbacks using DB, 15—20 reps
Seated concentration DB curls, 15—20 each arm
Repeat three to five times
Rest period 30—45 seconds

Circuit 4

Seated cable rows (machine), 12—15 reps
Standing triceps push-downs using tubing or bands, 12—15 reps
Standing bicep curls, 12—15 reps
Repeat three to five times
Rest period 30—45 seconds

At the end of your upper body workout, proceed to the abdominal circuit.

NAKED Tip

Don't compare your level of strength and ability with others. Love yourself as you are and work to reach your personal best.

NAKED Tip

Measure success by the way your clothes fit, your energy level or your reduction in pain or injury. Don't focus on a number on a scale. Most are not accurate anyway, and they say nothing about your overall health.

NAKED Tip

There is no accurate measurement or timetable to seeing results, but you can generally feel results happening on Day One. If you are sore, results are happening. As your body adapts to exercise, you are making internal changes, and that means results are happening. How well your body adapts to an exercise routine varies with every single individual, which is why you don't need to weigh yourself all the time. Some people start seeing results in a few days. Others may take many weeks. But none of that matters because the healthy lifestyle is what you are aiming for in the end.

Meal 1 (pre-workout)

Protein smoothie

1 scoop of protein powder shaken with 8 oz. of water.

NAKED Tip

Grocery shopping can be a meltdown if you're not prepared with a strategy. My top tips: never shop hungry, always bring a shopping list and don't veer from it, and stick to the perimeter, this is where the fruits and veggies live, as well as the dairy, meat and fish.

NAKED Tip

You rarely hear people talk about macadamia nuts, but macadamia nuts are packed with iron, calcium, magnesium and zinc. They are also rich in many B complex vitamins.

NAKED Tip

If you choose to have oatmeal for breakfast, top it with some chopped nuts like walnuts or almonds, and raisins or blueberries. Add a teaspoon of cinnamon for even more flavor.

NAKED Tip

My Mexican burrito: scrambled eggs with sliced peppers and onions. To a whole-grain tortilla, add the scrambled eggs, mashed up black beans and some spicy salsa.

Meal 2 (post-workout)

2 whole eggs, 1 egg white (cage free), 1 oz. baby spinach, 1 tsp coconut oil to make omelet; ⅛ tsp sea salt

½ avocado

NAKED Tip

Exercise is not just about spending an hour a day in the gym, walking or even doing yoga; it's a lifestyle of movement. Movement keeps your muscles toned, pumps oxygen through your bloodstream, fights bone frailty, flushes excess cholesterol, strengthens the immune system and helps keep you in a good mood. So bottom line: keep moving!

Meal 3 (lunch salad with a protein)

1½ cup mixed greens, spinach, baby spinach, baby kale, or a mix of both

6—8 oz. of lean meat

¼ cup of slivered almonds

1 tbsp. of dressing

NAKED Tip

A fan wrote that she loves this snack mid-day: 1 cup of mashed-up banana sprinkled with finely chopped almonds.

Meal 4 (snack)

1 rice cake with 1 tbsp. raw peanut butter or raw almond butter spread on top.

NAKED Tip

Studies show organically grown produce contains more vitamins, minerals and phytonutrients. Organic food is also free from pesticides and chemical residues that have been linked to nausea, headaches, vomiting and many serious medical conditions.

Meal 5 (dinner)

6—8 oz. salmon

Small side salad (e.g. 1 cup or less of spinach or kale) with chopped tomatoes and dressing

NAKED Tip

Garlic is known to increase the body's metabolic rate and this makes losing weight easier. It is also packed with flavor, using it makes withholding from using higher-calorie substitutes like butter easier to do.

Meal 6 (optional, can replace another meal or be a snack)

¼ cup of nuts

½ cup of berries

or

1 cup of popcorn, no butter, okay to season with a tbsp. herbs or spices

½ cup of berries

or
1 rice cake with 1 tbsp. of raw peanut butter or almond butter
¼ cup of berries

NAKED Tip

Studies have shown that people who take CoQ10, an over-the-counter supplement commonly available in pill form, regularly lose more weight because CoQ10 increases cellular energy so you burn more calories.

Mind/Spirit Tip: Have No Fear

In 2011, when I took on the tall task of scaling Mt. Kilimanjaro, my idea of camping was a weekend at the Four Seasons with room service and a spa. Climb the highest freestanding mountain in the world? I'd rather take the elevator.

What changed? How did a novice outdoorswoman conquer her fear of the outdoors, then a mountain? I started by turning it into a challenge. I've always loved a good challenge. If one person doubts that I can do something, it's a surefire way to get my butt in gear. Armed with the motivation I needed, my next task was to gather information.

Daniel Dorr's book *Kissing Kilimanjaro: Leaving It All on Top of Africa* had the answers I needed. The author explained step-by-step how he navigated the climb, including all the uncomfortable details about getting sick and getting frostbite. After reading the book, I felt prepared. The organizers of the climb gave me all the equipment I would need six months in advance. There were no secrets. I knew physically I could do it; now I was mentally prepared as well.

I've made a living helping improve people's physical fitness. From my experience, the hesitation to undertake a physical task—anything from a 30-day exercise program to climbing a 19,000-foot mountain—begins with the same fear that prevents us from undertaking more common tasks too. Public speaking is frequently cited as one of the most common, universal fears. *Project Runway* mentor Tim Gunn, on his first day as a teacher at the Parsons School of Design, was so afraid that he threw up before class. The singer Adele refused to play large arenas for years because of her fear of large crowds. Sarah Michelle Gellar has a fear of cemeteries, which was a big problem when she portrayed the title character in the television show *Buffy the Vampire Slayer.*

The point is, butterflies are butterflies. As a bodybuilder, I'd get butterflies every time I competed. My mouth would start to get dry whenever I heard my name called to the stage. The key is learning how to control it. For me, that meant turning every fear into a challenge, rehearsing the moment in my mind before it arrived and gathering all the information I needed until I was both mentally and physically prepared for the task in front of me. Think of fear as an emotion, just like love or happiness. You probably wouldn't confess you're in love after a first date, no matter how well it went. That's because you've learned how to control your expression of love and happiness. Fear shouldn't be any different.

If fear does make you physically ill, don't beat yourself up. It might just be in your head. There was once a high school teacher in Tennessee who complained of a "gasoline-like" smell in her classroom and became sick. Several students in the class felt similar symptoms, followed by the whole school. The building was evacuated and 38 people were hospitalized overnight. To everyone's surprise, the source of the smell was never identified. According to *The New England Journal of Medicine*, the outbreak was caused by something called "mass psychogenic illness." The cause of the outbreak was the fear of infection itself.

Remember that the next time you're feeling anxiety over an upcoming conversation, task or event. It's normal to feel sick or get butterflies. Turn it into a challenge and take baby steps to prepare. Maybe, as Franklin Roosevelt once said, "The only thing we have to fear is fear itself."

Day Twenty-Four

"If you fell down yesterday, stand up today."
—H.G. Wells

You're already halfway through the workout week. You should be feeling jazzed for your cardio workout today.

Go for a nice long run. Running not only helps me physically, it also helps me mentally. Once I started running, my confidence began to grow and I felt more in control of my life and my body.

Do your abs circuit and remember that you want to work up to three sets of 20 of each ab exercise. Push yourself to do one or two more crunches than you did yesterday.

NAKED Tip

Running relieves stress and anxiety. It boasts the brain's serotonin levels, which makes you calmer and more relaxed.

NAKED Tip

Don't aim for perfection with each and every workout. If you miss a workout, don't beat yourself up. Instead, consider it a rest day and get back to it the next day. If you find yourself unable to stick to your goals, simply reassess them. It's better to work out at a lower intensity or for less time for a while than not at all.

NAKED Tip

To help regulate your heart rate after a cardio workout, take the time to cool down. So many people are crunched for time and often want to skip the cool down. However, a cool down is designed primarily to help you slow your heart rate and lengthen muscle fibers that have been contracted during your workout. This action enhances your body's ability to recover beyond what it will do naturally, and your heart rate will follow suit.

Meal 1 (pre-workout)

Protein smoothie
1 scoop of protein powder shaken with 8 oz. of water.

NAKED Tip

Coconut milk also comes in a "lite" form. You can sauté chicken or even vegetables in lite coconut oil for curry.

Meal 2 (post-workout)

2 whole eggs, 1 egg white (cage free), 1 oz. baby spinach, 1 tsp coconut oil to make omelet; ⅛ tsp sea salt

NAKED Tip

Your health and your sleep habits are one. If you are having trouble sleeping, the lack of sleep will increase pain levels if you have joint or back pain and literally interfere with the regularity of every bodily function. Keep a good book by your bedside so that you can read if you can't sleep or you wake up, and if you wake up and simply cannot fall back asleep, get up and go to another room and read something relaxing, or take notes in a journal to note your patterns until you feel drowsy.

Meal 3 (lunch salad with a protein)

1 can of white tuna in water
1 cup mix of chopped broccoli, cauliflower, red onion and celery
Mix ¼ cup of olive oil with 3 tablespoons lemon juice, 2 tablespoons soy sauce, 1 tsp mustard.

NAKED Tip

Cherries don't get enough publicity for their amazing health benefits. They contain powerful antioxidants, reduce inflammation, reduce arthritis pain, reduce belly fat, and lower the risk of stroke to name just a few.

Meal 4 (snack)

2 celery stalks with raw peanut butter or raw almond butter

NAKED Tip

Vitamin D helps fight against diabetes and is a vitamin most people are deficient in because we simply do not spend enough time outside. The best source of vitamin D is direct sunlight, but that is not always an option for many of us. To naturally get more vitamin D in your diet, these foods can help: eggs, fish oil, anchovies, cod, shrimp, wild salmon and liver.

Meal 5 (dinner)

6—8 oz. lean turkey

1 cup of boiled broccoli, Brussels sprouts or cauliflower

NAKED Tip

Beet roots are edible and delicious. You can prepare these by sautéing beet greens with olive oil and garlic for a tasty side dish.

Meal 6 (optional, can replace another meal or be a snack)

¼ cup of nuts

½ cup of berries

or

1 cup of popcorn, no butter, okay to season with a tbsp. herbs or spices

½ cup of berries

or

1 rice cake with 1 tbsp. of raw peanut butter or almond butter

¼ cup of berries

NAKED Tip

Another great way to prepare beets is to bake them in the oven until they are soft, drizzle with some extra-virgin olive oil and sprinkle with some sea salt.

Mind/Spirit Tip: Spend Time Outdoors

I've lost count of how many gyms I belong to. I have a personal trainer too, plus a gym inside my home. I have access to every piece of equipment on the face of the earth. But the one thing I love more than anything is to be outside, in nature, with the fresh air and the birds chirping and the sky above my head. Gray sky, pouring rain—whatever—I love being outdoors for so many reasons.

I'll go deep on the dangers of smartphone use tomorrow. For today, remember it's important to leave your device at home whenever you take off power walking or running outdoors. It's therapeutic. Your phone won't blow up and, depending on where you are, no one can bother you. Even if your closest option is Manhattan's Central Park, there's something empowering about being in the presence of nature, if only for a moment. In those moments, I probably hash out over three-fourths of my issues, burdens and unresolved problems that I'm stuck on. It's the perfect time to sort through whatever is running through your head.

For me, that means no music too. I love a good album as much as anyone, but sometimes "silence is golden" (to quote an old song). Leave the earbuds next to your phone and go one-on-one with your thoughts and problems. You'll find being in touch with nature is a great way to be in touch with yourself.

Science has my back on this too. Harvard University's health department offers several good reasons to get outdoors:

1. Sunlight hitting your skin begins a process that leads to the creation and activation of vitamin D, which is believed to combat everything from osteoporosis and cancer to depression and heart attacks.
2. You'll get more exercise. Stepping outside more should mean less time in front of the television and computer, and more time walking and doing other things that put your body in motion.
3. Light tends to elevate your mood, and there's usually more light available outdoors than in. Physical activity has been shown to help people relax and cheer up.
4. Your concentration will improve. Children with ADHD seem to focus better after being outdoors. Maybe you don't have ADHD, but try stepping outside if you're having trouble concentrating. It can't hurt.
5. One study showed that people recovering from spinal surgery experienced less pain and stress, and took fewer pain

> medications, when they were exposed to natural light. Another study showed that hospital patients whose window faced a tree recovered faster than those whose window faced a brick wall.

So, how much time should you spend outdoors every day? Twenty minutes is enough to significantly boost a person's vitality levels, according to one study. The same study found that even imagining yourself in a natural setting can improve your energy. Keep that in mind the next time you're stuck at the office and can't duck outside for a while. It's a great alternative to coffee!

Can't get out during the daytime? Try sunset. On the island of Santorini, a popular destination in the Aegean Sea, watching the sun set is a daily ritual. People gather on the coast to get a glimpse and take pictures, then applaud once the sun dips below the horizon. It's also a spiritual experience, if only a little touristy—and a great mental snapshot to boost your energy the next time you close your eyes at work.

It's also a reminder that no matter where you go, whether for business or for pleasure, nature goes with you. You can always poke your head outdoors.

Day Twenty-Five

"I have walked that long road to freedom. I have tried not to falter; I have made missteps along the way. But I have discovered the secret that after climbing a great hill, one only finds that there are many more hills to climb. I have taken a moment here to rest, to steal a view of the glorious vista that surrounds me, to look back on the distance I have come. But I can only rest for a moment, for with freedom come responsibilities, and I dare not linger, for my long walk is not ended."

—Nelson Mandela

Regular lower-body exercise increases bone strength, improves your balance and stamina, and decreases the injury risk to your knees and hips, along with your risk of falling. Also, a strong lower body helps slow the physical weakness that is part of the aging process and maintains balance, stamina and confidence.

Today is your last lower-body routine of my 30-day program. Be sure to begin with the hamstring glute stretch to get your muscles warmed up and ready to go.

Drink plenty of water and don't forget to complete your workout with the abdominal circuit.

Lower-body circuit (45 to 60 minutes)

Five-minute warm-up

Leg extensions 15—20 reps four sets

Circuit 1

Smith machine squats, 15—20 reps

Walking lunges, 50 to 75 yards

Seated or kneeling leg curls machine, 15—20 reps

Repeat three or four sets
Rest period 30—45 seconds

Circuit 2

Seated leg press (machine), 15—20 reps
Standing body weight squats, 30—40 reps
Anterior reach lunge, 12—15 each leg
Repeat four to five times
Rest period 30—45 seconds

Circuit 3

Jump squats, 30 seconds
Alternating jumping lunges, 30 seconds
Repeat three to four times
Rest period 30—45 seconds

Circuit 4

Lying glute bridge off stability ball, legs straight, 15—20 reps
Lying glute bridge with knees bent, feet flat on ball, pushing hips up as high as you can, 15—20 reps
Lying leg curls on stability ball 15—20 reps
Repeat three to four times
Rest period 30—45 seconds

NAKED Tip

Make the assumption that you are going to feel sore for the first few weeks of any workout program. Don't go all out on the first day or even the first week. Ramp things up each day based on how you feel. If you do feel sore, back off a little, but don't stop. Doing a workout at 50 percent is a lot better than doing nothing at all. It will also help your soreness fade quicker.

NAKED Tip

Stay safe during your workouts. Although I talk throughout this book about increasing your intensity and your amount of reps, you should never push yourself to the point of injury. Challenging your body helps your fitness improve and progress, but don't overdo it. Be smart. You want to stay healthy and safe throughout the program.

NAKED Tip

You should always lift as much weight as you can for the number of repetitions targeted by an exercise. If you aren't doing this, you're only tapping a fraction of your workout's potential. You'll achieve the most gains by pushing your body to its limit. You should barely make the last rep of every set, which is impossible to do unless you fail on occasion to determine your progress. So while failure is never your goal, it's also not an option when you're trying your hardest. It will happen sometimes, and, when it does, you'll know you're on the right track.

Meal 1 (pre-workout)

Protein smoothie

1 scoop of protein powder shaken with 8 oz. of water.

NAKED Tip

Swiss chard is amazing vegetable that comes in these gorgeous multi-colored stems and veins, sometimes called "rainbow chard." They are packed with vitamins and antioxidant properties and can be simply sautéed or steamed and tossed with a nice vinaigrette.

Meal 2 (post-workout)

Awesome omelet

1 large egg

4 egg whites

½ tsp. sea salt

1 tablespoon freshly chopped cilantro

¼ cup chopped onion

¼ cup black beans

¼ cup tomatoes

Meal 3 (lunch salad with a protein)

1 can of white tuna in water

1 cup mix of chopped broccoli, cauliflower, red onion and celery

Mix ¼ cup of olive oil with 3 tablespoons lemon juice, 2 tablespoons soy sauce, 1 tsp mustard.

NAKED Tip

Collard greens are more popular in the South and contain a wealth of vitamins, most prominently K and C, folate and beta-carotene. The easiest way to prepare them is to boil them in water, drain and chop to add to salads or top with a lean chicken or turkey.

Meal 4 (snack)

2 celery stalks with raw peanut butter or raw almond butter

NAKED Tip

Peas are good for your digestion and help lower cholesterol levels. Boil or microwave peas for salads, alone, or in soups.

Meal 5 (dinner)

6—8 oz. flank steak, cooked to taste
1½ cup baby kale
1 cup chopped tomatoes
Salt and pepper to taste

NAKED Tip

Don't underestimate the power of beef. Protein is what helps build muscles, boost your immune system and heal wounds. It also helps carry oxygen to the blood cells to prevent muscle fatigue.

Meal 6 (optional, can replace another meal or be a snack)

¼ cup of nuts
½ cup of berries
or
1 cup of popcorn, no butter, okay to season with a tbsp. herbs or spices
½ cup of berries
or
1 rice cake with 1 tbsp. of raw peanut butter or almond butter
¼ cup of berries

NAKED Tip

A fan wrote to me that he makes his own almond butter in a food processor and just adds a little honey. Because almonds are so nutritionally dense, you get more vitamins and minerals from them than any other nut for every calorie consumed.

Mind/Spirit Tip: Put Away Your Phone

Smartphones, and technology in general, come with the promise of making our lives easier. To an extent they do. It's nice not having to find a payphone anymore (remember those?), then a quarter, then the person's phone number, when you want to place a call outside your house.

Text messaging is convenient. I use smartphone apps for banking, sending and receiving email and listening to music. That's about it. Sure, there are apps to tell you how much you're sleeping and how many calories you've eaten or burned. There are also apps that indulge bad habits, like ordering all sorts of unhealthy food. Good or bad, for the life of me I can't remember an app I can't live without.

For many of you, however, technology addiction is complicating your life in ways you can't understand. Millennials are more forgetful than seniors now. Studies have shown that on average, we spend about one-third of our waking hours checking our mobile devices. As a result, we're more moody, lonely and jealous. Maybe it was Arianna Huffington—ironically, the founder of one of the most heavily trafficked news websites in the world—who put it best: "So often, especially now with this addiction to technology, we find ourselves so disconnected from ourselves that we don't know who we are."

The purpose of this book isn't simply to feel better naked when you look in a mirror. It's about getting naked emotionally and spiritually and not feeling ashamed of what you see on the inside too. Any addiction, whether it's to shopping or drugs or technology, will separate us from our naked self. It hides the people we were put on the planet to be. For some of you, the very thing you're addicted to might be sitting in your pocket right now.

The smartphone can do some powerful, scary stuff to your brain. Journalist Nicholas Carr, in his book *The Shallows: How the Internet Is Changing the Way We Think, Read and Remember,* argues that the cost of being constantly inundated with information is our ability to be contemplative and engage in the kind of deep thinking that requires us to concentrate on one thing. One recent study asked participants to estimate the amount of time they spend on their phone, then compared their self-reports to actual usage. The results: the average person checked their device 85 times a day—twice as often as they thought—totaling five hours using apps and surfing the web. No wonder we can't concentrate anymore!

Maybe because we can't concentrate, our brains tend to give up. Research has shown that high-volume smartphone users let their phones, in essence, take up thinking on their behalf. They also score lower on certain cognitive tests. The phenomenon is particularly true for people who rely more on intuition than analytical thought.

Most friends my age don't seem to be battling with technology to the same degree as our children's generation. I can still remember taking typing classes in high school—and hating it. That was one of my early battles with technology. But if your job demands that you be glued to the Internet, or your phone or your iPad at all hours, it's important to know the byproducts of constant connection. You're increasing your exposure to stress, mitigating your immune system and digestion and putting yourself in danger of losing touch with yourself.

If that sounds like you, take time out of each day to go device-free. Figure out how much time you have to disconnect—10 minutes, a half-hour, an hour—and commit to doing it every day. There are plenty of suggestions in these pages for what to do with all that time. Trust me, it's healthier than staring at a screen.

Day Twenty-Six

"Two roads diverged in a wood, and I— / I took the one less traveled by / And that has made all the difference."

—Robert Frost

You should be feeling exuberant today! If you've been following my program all along, your energy levels should be off the charts. You're well on your way to getting in the best shape of your life and it's very likely you are even yearning for your workout today.

Increase the intensity of your cardio workout today by taking a fitness class like Zumba, which burns 400 calories per hour, or a Soul Cycle class (if there's one near you) a super-fast-paced spin class with a club-like vibe. You might even want to try a bootcamp workout, which is an excellent way to get in shape and take your fitness to the next level.

Do your abs routine and give yourself a high five when you're done!

NAKED Tip

Feeling burned out? Don't focus on what you haven't achieved yet. Focus on the good stuff. Celebrate your daily successes. Take at least one minute every day to journal one fitness achievement. It may be that you completed the entire set of an exercise for the first time that you trained even though you really didn't feel like it, or that you hit the amount of reps you were aiming for.

NAKED Tip

Great abs is not only the ultimate symbol of being fit and lean, but a strong core helps stabilize your entire body. To get the most out of your abs workout, try to incorporate more core work into your workout schedule. Core training increases your overall functional fitness, so you won't just look better but you'll be able to function better as a whole.

NAKED Tip

If you use your workout gear past its expiration point, you could be doing your body more harm than good, so it becomes important to understand how long your shoes might last and how to know when it's time to shop for new ones. When it comes to shoes, you tend to get what you pay for. Shoes that are purpose-designed with higher-quality materials tend to last longer. But no matter the manufacturer, studies have shown most shoes exhibit similar wear in one very important area: compression capabilities, or their ability to absorb the shock of you jumping. The best way to know if your shoes are done is to do a visual inspection of the shoe itself. Don't just look on the underside of the shoe. Take the time to inspect areas that display wear and tear long before, such as the midsole, which is visible from the side of the shoe. If the midsole shows excessive horizontal creasing or wear on the areas that absorb the most load—the heel and the ball of the foot—then it's probably time to toss them.

Meal 1 (pre-workout)

Protein smoothie

1 scoop of protein powder shaken with 8 oz. of water.

NAKED Tip

Adding ground cinnamon to a protein shake is a great way to get that cinnamon bun flavor.

Meal 2 (post-workout)

2 eggs, 1 egg white (cage-free) for scrambled eggs or omelet with:

¼ cup chopped red onion

½ chopped green pepper

⅓ cup spinach

NAKED Tip

If you like peppermint, another great way to add kick to your protein shake is to add a tsp. of peppermint extract.

Meal 3 (lunch salad with a protein)

6—8 oz. grilled skinless chicken breast

1½ cup mixed greens, spinach, baby spinach, baby kale, or a mix of both

¼ cup of slivered almonds

1 tbsp. of dressing

NAKED Tip

Kale is not the only vegetable you can crisp. Slice up some parsnips, carrots, beets, yucca or taro root, and place them in the oven on a cookie sheet. Sprinkle with extra virgin olive oil and bake until crisp. I also like to slice *all* of these and mix it up—it is also very colorful.

Meal 4 (snack)

1—2 cups of kale to make crispy kale chips

Spread raw kale leaves on a cookie sheet sprayed with olive oil

Drizzle 1 tbsp of olive oil over the kale leaves and top with pinch of sea salt

Cook at 375 degrees until crispy

NAKED Tip

Add sugar snap peas to your snack list. They're water soluble, high in vitamin C and help boost the immune system among so many other benefits. Buy a bag or bunch in the grocery store and eat them cold. The cold and the crunch will really hold you over.

Meal 5 (dinner)

6—8 oz. grilled skinless chicken breasts, sliced into strips

1—2 cups mixed greens

¼ red onion, sliced in long, thin slices

½ cup black beans

1 tablespoon dressing.

NAKED Tip

If you like slaw, try one with just carrots and parsnips. Drizzle with oil and vinegar and sprinkle with salt and pepper to taste.

Meal 6 (optional, can replace another meal or be a snack)

¼ cup of nuts

½ cup of berries

or

1 cup of popcorn, no butter, okay to season with a tbsp. herbs or spices

½ cup of berries

or

1 rice cake with 1 tbsp. of raw peanut butter or almond butter

¼ cup of berries

NAKED Tip

Here's an awesome summer salad: chunks of cucumber, tomato and red onion with a balsamic vinaigrette dressing. So simple and so delicious.

Mind/Spirit Tip: Live with No Regrets

Regret nothing. It makes for a great T-shirt slogan, but can a person really live with no regrets?

Think about it this way. We have two choices in life. We can either set goals, try to achieve them and sometimes fail in the process, or we can never try and never fail. Which of the two choices leads to a life of no regrets?

At some point in my 40s I decided the never-try, never-fail policy wasn't for me. I realized failures and mistakes are simply a way of learning life's lessons. If you go through life without making a mistake or failing at something, there was no lesson learned, no wisdom gained. All those failures and missteps that weigh on your conscience don't have to be regrets or anything that raises your blood pressure at all. They're actually a way forward.

I can only wish I was born with that insight, or learned it at an early age. Quite the contrary, I was raised in a home that was emotionally, mentally and physically abusive. My siblings and I were often told we were good for nothing. We were never told we were loved. I was the victim of mind games, manipulations, broomsticks, belts and kicks. When I was small enough, I was stuffed into a cupboard. During my first marriage, I was physically and mentally abused again. By the time I left my first husband at age 25, I felt as though I didn't deserve to breathe the same air as everyone else.

Maybe you've experienced the pain of divorce too. That's a time when it's only natural to experience a sense of regret about your circumstances. But just because a marriage ends in a divorce doesn't mean you'll never remarry. Own your mistakes, learn from them and make progress. That way the next chapter in your life won't be a repeat of the last. Think of your life as a book. The fewer chapters you repeat, the less likely you are to feel regret.

Psychologists define regret as "a negative cognitive/emotional state that involves blaming ourselves for a bad outcome, feeling a sense of loss or sorrow at what might have been, or wishing we could undo a previous choice that we made." What a sad drain on our energy! To be fully unclothed emotionally, we need to bury our regrets in the past. Maybe that means forgiving yourself or asking someone for forgiveness. Maybe that means apologizing to someone. As much as anything, that means living in the present. I've devoted one section in this book to each of these critical skills.

And how far can living in the present take a person? Consider the case of Donald Trump, who filed for Chapter 11 bankruptcy four times in a span of 19 years. Rather than dwelling on the regret of his failed businesses, what did Trump do? He ran for president—twice!

Some of you might feel a sense of pride when someone you haven't seen in a while says you haven't changed a bit. Not me. I consider it a compliment whenever I hear, "Theresa, you're so different than you were ten years ago." I was a mess ten years ago, still reeling from the death of my son. I wouldn't want to stay a mess for ten years. Growth and change is a good thing, and it comes from mistakes and failures.

Regretting nothing is a choice within your power—and a great choice at that!

Day Twenty-Seven

"Twenty years from now you will be more disappointed by the things that you didn't do than by the ones you did do, so throw off the bowlines, sail away from safe harbor, catch the trade winds in your sails. Explore, Dream, Discover."
—Mark Twain

You've made it to your last upper-body strength-training workout of the week. By now, you know all the benefits that strength training has to offer your body now and in the future. Keep your strength-training goals at the forefront of your mind as you go through the circuit today. It will help motivate you to the next level of your workout.

NAKED Tip

Lifting weights increases functional fitness, which makes everyday tasks such as carrying children, lifting grocery bags and picking up heavy suitcases much easier. According to the Mayo Clinic, regular weight training can make you 50 percent stronger in six months. Being strong is also empowering. Not only does it improve your physical activities, it builds emotional strength by boosting self-esteem and confidence.

NAKED Tip

The more you work your entire body, the better it is for your abs. Most exercises, from push-ups to squats to deadlifts, require a lot of ab effort. Working your full body will burn many more calories and raise your metabolism, which is important, because you also need to lose fat to make your abs flat. When you combine an effective full-body workout with a proper diet, like my NAKED Program, getting the abs you've always wanted is just a matter of time.

NAKED Tip

Wearing a good sports bra can make all the difference in the world when you're working out. If you're on the small side, you can probably get enough support from a basic compression bra, which is super supportive. If you're more endowed, look for an encapsulation bra, which keeps your breasts in separate cups. You can even layer bras for extra support. The great news is that fitness fashion has come such a long way, so have fun shopping for your favorite brands when looking for the right support.

Meal 1 (pre-workout)

Protein smoothie

1 scoop of protein powder shaken with 8 oz. of water.

NAKED Tip:

Another great go-to snack: mash up some chickpeas and spread the mash over stalks of celery. You have the crunch with the creamy and only good ingredients.

Meal 2 (post-workout)

¼ cup cream of rice cereal mixed in 1 cup of water

Boil the rice/water mixture in the microwave for about three minutes. If you use more water, the mixture is more watery like farina; less water and it's chunkier like a pudding.

1 tsp of cinnamon sprinkled on top

Pinch of sea salt

NAKED Tip

Can you imagine a chickpea cookie dough? Yep, there is such a thing and many people love it. Mash up ½ cup chickpeas and add ¼ cup or less of chocolate chips.

Meal 3 (lunch salad with a protein)

1½ cup mixed greens, spinach, baby spinach, baby kale, or a mix of both

6—8 oz. of lean meat

¼ cup of slivered almonds

1 tbsp. of dressing

NAKED Tip

I love to have a bag of edamame for dinner. You can buy edamame in the shells in the frozen foods section of the grocery store and simply microwave for about three minutes. They come up steamy and delicious. Sprinkle some sea salt on top. You can also buy bags of edamame out of the pods and roast them in the oven with a little garlic and salt. Edamame is filled with fiber and a good muscle-building protein.

Meal 4 (snack)

1 rice cake with 1 tbsp. raw peanut butter or raw almond butter spread on top.

NAKED Tip

Spinach and kale with chopped up strawberries and walnuts is a great, quick summer salad you might not expect. Chop and toss everything evenly with a vinaigrette.

Meal 5 (dinner)

6—8 oz. of salmon

Small side salad (e.g. 1 cup or less of spinach or kale) with chopped tomatoes and dressing

NAKED Tip

Shrimp boils typically consist of shrimp, corn on the cob, red skin potatoes and sausage. Simply remove the sausage and steam the shrimp, corn on the cob and some chopped up parsnips. Add Old Bay Seasoning to taste. Parsnips are very high in fiber and a good replacement for potatoes in a shrimp boil.

Meal 6 (optional, can replace another meal or be a snack)

¼ cup of nuts

½ cup of berries

or

1 cup of popcorn, air popped and no butter, okay to season with a tbsp. herbs or spices

½ cup of berries

or

1 rice cake with 1 tbsp. of raw peanut butter or almond butter

¼ cup of berries

NAKED Tip

Dr. Oz has said that he always has a few (5 to 7) almonds at night before he goes to bed because it's a nice snack. They have tremendous anti-inflammatory benefits.

Mind/Spirit Tip: Take a Vacation

Some of the strongest memories of my childhood are of summer vacations. The idea of spending time away from home with my family always brought excitement. Packing our bags and going away for a while was the one thing I truly looked forward to once school let out. Funny thing is, it didn't matter where we went. Whether camping in the woods, sleeping in a hotel or bunking on a farm, everyone pressed Pause on life to spend time together. It was great.

Just think about all the power meditating packs into a momentary vacation from your thoughts. Now imagine multiplying that moment out over a weekend or even a full week. No wonder we still need vacations as adults. They're essential to our mental and spiritual wellbeing.

The health-care conglomerate Health Net Inc. identifies specific benefits for working professionals who are thinking about taking a vacation. According to an internal study of Ernst & Young employees, for each additional ten hours of vacation employees took, their year-end performance ratings actually *improved* by eight percent. The Boston Consulting Group found that high-level professionals who were required to take time off were significantly more productive overall than those who spent more time working. Think you're too busy to take a vacation? Maybe you're too busy *not* to take a vacation!

The benefits extend beyond the workplace. According to Health Net, a study of 1,500 women in rural Wisconsin determined that those who vacationed less than once every two years were more likely to suffer from depression and increased stress than those who took vacations at least twice a year. Another study counted lower blood pressure, smaller waistlines, higher positive emotional levels and less depression among the benefits of vacationing.

The American Psychological Association recommends taking vacations to reduce stress levels, and we know too much stress is bad for your heart. It shouldn't surprise you to learn that women who reported taking a vacation once every six years or less are almost eight times more likely to develop coronary heart disease or have a heart attack compared to women who vacation at least twice a year.

Okay, you might be thinking, *I'll finally take that vacation I've been planning forever*. Just don't forget to put away your smartphone. Recall the power of powering down your screens. It can be particularly powerful on short vacations where you don't wander far from home. Depending on how often you use your favorite devices, merely turning them all off for a short period of time can be a vacation in itself.

It's critically important to be present when vacationing with children, because a lifelong memory is hanging in the balance. At a young age, the quality time *is* the vacation. A moment spent glued to your smartphone on vacation is a moment lost forever. That memory can linger long into adulthood. Never forget how important it is to keep the promise of a family vacation. There's nothing you can accomplish sitting by the pool glued to your iPad that's more important than a human interaction with your kids.

Wherever you go, vacating your busy life and buzzing phone will allow your mind, body and spirit—and your family—to reap the benefits long after you return. Still, go far from home when you can. Research shows that traveling abroad allows us to have a more nuanced understanding of ourselves and who we are. A physical journey can help you make the most of your personal journey too.

Day Twenty-Eight

"We will chase perfection and we will chase it relentlessly, knowing all the while we can never attain it. But along the way, we shall catch excellence."

—Vince Lombardi

Congratulations! You have reached the final rest day of my NAKED Program. You should feel elated and proud of yourself for committing to the program thus far and for what you have accomplished up to this point. Enjoy your rest day and celebrate you today. You deserve it.

NAKED Tip

Take a hot, steamy bubble bath on rest day. If you are experiencing sore muscles or aches, a bath may help to relax muscles and make the pain and discomfort more manageable. Sit back, relax and let your sore muscles recover.

NAKED Tip

If a hot, steamy bath doesn't work for you, try an ice bath, ice massage or contrast water therapy (alternating hot and cold showers) to recover faster, reduce muscle soreness and prevent injury. The theory behind this method is that repeatedly constricting and dilating blood vessels helps remove (or flush out) waste products in the tissues.

NAKED Tip

You've heard me mention that recovery after exercise is essential to muscle and tissue repair and strength building. This is even more critical after a heavy weight-training session. A muscle needs anywhere from 24—48 hours to repair and rebuild, and working it again too soon simply leads to tissue breakdown instead of building. It goes without saying that you should never work out the same muscle group two days in a row.

Mind/Spirit Tip: Eliminate Toxic Relationships

There's a person in my family who has to call my lawyer if he wants to talk to me. He knows this. He knows the terms of the restraining order against him. There's another person whose emails are filtered straight into my junk mail folder, whose phone number is blocked and whose hand-written letters go straight to my recycling bin. It saddens me to write this, so I take no pride in listing these facts. I'm just not proud of the people who forced me to eliminate them from my life.

Toxic relationships poison our lives by definition, to the point that everything they touch destroys a part of you. Toxic people are like a cancer. Sometimes their path of destruction creeps along little by little. Sometimes they act swiftly, knocking out an entire organ by consuming your thoughts. If you don't have any personal experience with a relationship so toxic, congratulations! Be grateful, and be prepared to act in case you do. If you have toxic people in your life currently, and you haven't taken whatever steps are necessary to improve your relationship or cut them off altogether, don't waste your time. Just as nothing can lift our minds and spirits quite like the love of another person, nothing can ruin your mind and spirit more than someone else too.

Eliminating toxic people from your life begins with the self-confidence to recognize you deserve better. Sadly, I didn't have that until I was in my 40s. From there, cutting someone off can be easy—a simple matter of ignoring them or a straightforward "please don't call, write or visit me again." Other times, well, get ready to fight.

Lawyers and restraining orders should be your last resort, a final ultimatum for someone who ignores your requests to stay away. In the case of my two family members, all the previous ultimatums didn't work. So where did I draw the line?

When my mother told me, "As far as I'm concerned, you're dead in my world," that was it. She was out.

When my stepson—who by then had defamed me, harassed me, and gone on the Internet to destroy my reputation and threaten my life—started causing sleepless nights and my husband's chest pain, that was it. He was out.

Again, I take no pleasure in telling these stories. Cutting family out of my life hurt my heart. But it hurt more to have them in my life. When someone is hurting you so much it affects your body, mind or spirit, don't be afraid to stick up for yourself. The short-term pain will be replaced with the sense of freedom that comes with feeling whole.

If that's something you've never felt, you'll have to trust me: don't waste another day with a toxic person. Sherry Gaba, an author and therapist who specializes in addictions, writes: "To the individual that is living in the [toxic] relationship, they can't imagine a healthy interaction with their significant other. In their mind, their interactions with their significant other are normal. What these individuals lack are proper keys to communication. They can't imagine a relationship that would be healthy, encouraging and sane."

Recovering from a toxic relationship takes time. Often, it requires professional help. Earlier, I explained the importance of asking for help. You might be on top of the world professionally and still have no clue how to forge a healthy relationship in your personal life. If that sounds like you, don't be ashamed. One poisonous person might be the only thing separating you from your most beautiful naked self.

Day Twenty-Nine

"Nothing will work unless you do."
—Maya Angelou

This is your last cardio workout of my program. By now you're body is craving the sweat and the high intensity. Choose a challenging workout that is worthy of your will and determination. Go all out. Beat it.

Kick that abs routine in the butt. You're well on your way to getting that toned tummy you've always wanted.

NAKED Tip

Taking a few extra minutes to clean up your workout gear can make the difference between healthy and sick. Whether you're at the gym or at home, be sure to clean your equipment, including weights, yoga mats and resistance bands with mild soapy water. With an increasing number of people being diagnosed with skin infections caused by *Staphylococcus aureus* ("staph") bacteria that are resistant to many antibiotics, there's no reason to take a chance, because no matter how much you love working out, there's nothing fun about catching a disease.

NAKED Tip

If you work out at home, you want to be able to create a comfortable space that will help motivate you to work out. Consider setting up your workout space in a part of the home that doesn't have a lot of traffic. For example, if you set up your home gym in the den, your workout time may conflict with when others want to watch TV—a battle you're likely to lose. Invest in the right workout equipment like dumbbells, resistance bands, a pull-up bar and workout bench. Also having the proper flooring in your workout space can make the difference between sore knees and healthy knees. If you're going to be jumping or doing exercises that may cause you to slip, put down a few locking rubber mats with rug runners beneath them so they don't slide. The padding will make the surface softer to land on and you shouldn't go flying.

By investing in the right equipment, selecting the best room and paying attention to the surface you're working out on, you can create the ultimate workout space that makes working out a pleasure, not a chore!

NAKED Tip

When it comes to getting the most out of your workouts, do it on an empty stomach, which can be anywhere from ten minutes to three hours, depending on the size of your meal. The general rule is to wait three hours after a full, balanced meal. Wait two hours after a lighter meal. Wait one hour after a snack. For anything less than an hour, keep your snack below 100 calories.

Mind/Spirit Tip: Dress For Success

You can't be naked all the time. As you eat better and exercise more, at some point you'll probably want—and maybe need—new clothes to fit the new shape of your new body. You've lived enough by now that hopefully you can judge the difference between clothes that accentuate your unique body and clothes that don't. (If you can't, well, that's another book for another time!) Not everyone will dress for success exactly the same way. The point here isn't to explain how to perfect your wardrobe, but rather how your wardrobe can affect your mind and spirit.

For the most part, this idea sounds intuitive. When you look good, you feel good. You're more likely to have a smile on your face when you're wearing a brand-new evening gown than your old sweatpants. Believe it or not, there are actually scientists who research the psychological effects of clothing—and not everything they discover is intuitive.

Here's one: wearing formal clothing in the workplace can help employees focus on big-picture ideas more than their casually-dressed colleagues. "Formal clothing," concluded one of the study's authors, "might improve your mood if you feel good in the clothing and think it looks good." Have you ever waitressed? Think about how it felt to put on that uniform, compared to the feeling at the end of a long day of slipping on a nice dress you chose for yourself. There's a reason prisoners are all given the same drab uniforms to wear. They're supposed to blend in, not feel empowered.

But how empowering can one piece of clothing be? A university professor once asked her students to put on Superman T-shirts, then gave them a survey. The students rated themselves as more likeable and superior than students who weren't wearing the T-shirts. They judged themselves to be physically stronger than they felt in their own clothing. There are no shortcuts to looking good naked, but at least the right clothes offer a temporary shortcut to self-esteem.

Besides focusing your mind and lifting your spirits, your clothes will affect how you're judged by other people. One study determined that your clothing affects how others perceive your competence, independence and creativity. Still another concluded that even the color of your clothes can cause another woman to guard her partner more closely. (Hint: red clothes signal to the world that you're on the prowl!) With all this subconscious judgment going on, how disheartening would it be if one poor choice in clothing undermined your excellent new choices in diet, exercise and lifestyle?

There's even a Biblical parable that jibes with the wisdom of these experiments. Jesus said that "no one puts new wine into old wineskins. If he does, the wine will burst the skins—and the wine is destroyed, so are the skins" (Mark 2:22). Jesus was making a point about shedding your old self in the process of inner transformation. For some of you, the same principle will apply to your clothes. Don't trap the new you inside an old outfit.

In *You Are What You Wear: What Your Clothes Reveal about You*, author and psychologist Jennifer Baumgartner writes, "when we shop for and wear clothing that reflects our best self, we must consider, consciously or unconsciously, our age, size, culture, and lifestyle. We either work with these aspects of ourselves or fight against them." When you look good and feel good naked, it should shine through when you're wearing clothes too.

Day Thirty

"The challenge is not to be perfect… it's to be whole."
—Jane Fonda

I want to personally thank you for taking me on this 30-day journey with you. I hope you have learned a lot about yourself and have reached your goals. For some of you, 30 days is just the beginning, and I hope you'll continue to allow me to help you reach your goals.

For those of you who like what you see when you look in the mirror and want to continue getting in the best shape of your life, this is the first day of the rest of your journey.

Complete your upper-body strength-training workout while you visualize your finish line.

NAKED Tip

Adding a mental practice to your workout routine can be a huge benefit for anyone. Spending time following a mindfulness meditation program can help process a calm, clear attitude and reduce anxiety and reactivity. Getting familiar with how your mind works, how thoughts can bounce around and how you don't need to attach to any of them, is a wonderful way for an athlete to recover both mentally and physically. Additionally, practicing positive self-talk with a can-do attitude can help change the ongoing dialogue in your head. Consider using both types of mental practice during your recovery days.

NAKED Tip

Strength-training programs require constant adjustment, or you may find yourself stuck in a rut and hitting a plateau. That is why I have encouraged you to switch things up during your workouts. If you are new to strength training, you may find you get stronger fairly quickly, then suddenly, you find yourself in a holding pattern. To continue making gains you have to vary your training techniques and understand basic conditioning. One way to break a training plateau is by making your muscles work harder, rather than longer. At this point in your training you should try "high weight—low reps" rather than "low weight—high reps." If you had been lifting three sets of 12—15 reps with 5 lbs., drop down to one set of 6—8 reps with 8 lbs.

NAKED Tip

Most people become frustrated and quit exercising before they see any real results. But it's not too surprising, given the common mistakes many people make with their training programs. These tips will help you stick to your program and achieve your goals:

- Focus on what you're doing and increase the quality of every movement. Once you start exercising with a real purpose, and pushing both your aerobic capacity and your strength, you will find your workouts take half the time.
- Set realistic goals. Be honest with yourself about your abilities, your level of commitment and your lifestyle. Then set appropriate goals that start from where you are and progress at a reasonable rate.
- Many people are in denial about the foods they eat, and particularly, the quantity consumed. If you really want to lose weight, you need to be honest with yourself about what you put into your mouth and how that helps or hinders your weight-loss goals. To get real with yourself, write it down. Tracking what you eat in a food diary will help you break the cycle of food denial.

Mind/Spirit Tip: Be Yourself and Don't Apologize

So you're having fun. You're meditating. You're exercising, you're feeling better, and you're getting better in touch with your naked self. Here's the thing: not everyone will like this. The world isn't full of cheerleaders. There will be people, even friends, who resent your success and want you to be more like them—not because they don't want you to look and feel your best, but because they suddenly feel inferior when they're around you. At some point, you might be tempted to apologize.

My advice: don't. This isn't just a nugget of wisdom to apply in the spur of a heated moment, though it's that too. Owning who you are, and taking pride in your transformation, is an important component of your mental and spiritual wellbeing in the long run. There's a proper way to respond to those who resent our successes and those who delight in our failures. Apologizing just isn't it.

At some point, every one of us *will* encounter a situation where it's appropriate to apologize to someone else. In those times, it's important to be mindful about what we're apologizing for. One thing we should never apologize for is being ourselves. Caitlyn Jenner, who lived for 65 years as a man named Bruce, is a perfect example of what I mean.

As a public figure—first as an Olympic champion, then a television personality—Jenner was forced to live a lie in front of millions. As a woman, she faced criticism for her appearance. Gender dysphoria is an unusual, extreme condition. Many will find it hard to see their own struggle reflected in Caitlyn Jenner. Yet if you've ever been wrongly criticized for how you look, how you talk or how you act, it shouldn't be too hard to relate. Until you know another person's story, it really isn't fair to criticize them.

People have criticized me assuming that I grew up wealthy, for having a 3,000 square foot closet in my home filled with designer goods and for dressing like a younger woman. When tuning out the critics, it helps to have a reservoir of confidence. It also helped, in my case, that the criticism was simply not true. I did not grow up wealthy. I've used my big closet space for charity functions and auctioning off its contents. The way I dress reflects the age I feel, not the age on my driver's license—and I encourage everyone to do the same! None of these things demand an apology. You probably don't have to dig too deep to find a similar example from your own life.

We've all been in the other person's shoes, too. Sometimes the temptation to criticize others is hard to resist. When I was a fitness instructor I was surrounded by different people with different stories. Many came to my class to escape their troubles. My job, beyond smiling and giving exercise instructions, was to provide a respite. One student in particular always arrived to class looking upset, and she often took out her frustration on me. Until I knew her story, I couldn't help but take it personally. After we finally talked it over, we became friends.

It took me years to learn not to apologize for simply being myself. Too often I see people who haven't grasped this important life lesson. Remember, you're not living your life for other people. Before we can begin filling up that internal reservoir of confidence, we must accept that not everyone will like us for who we are. That's an unrealistic expectation. Letting go of that expectation will result in fewer apologies. It might be the best trade you ever make.

Appendix A

SPARTA FITNESS

NAME: AGE: TRAINER:

Date:		Height:		Weight:	

Caliper Measurements

Chest:		Suprillac:		Bicep:	
Subscap:		Thigh:		Calf:	
Abd:		Low Bck:		Tricep:	

Girth Measurements

Shoulders:		Chest:		Waist:		Hips:		L.Bi:	
L Thigh:		R.Thigh:		L.Calf:		R.Calf:		R.Bi:	

Body Fat%:		
Fat Lbs:		
Lean Mass:		

Date:		Weight:			

Caliper Measurements

Chest:		Suprillac:		Bicep:	
Subscap:		Thigh:		Calf:	
Abd:		Low Bck:		Tricep:	

Girth Measurements

Shoulders:		Chest:		Waist:		Hips:		L.Bi:	
L Thigh:		R.Thigh:		L.Calf:		R.Calf:		R.Bi:	

Body Fat%:		
Fat Lbs:		
Lean Mass:		

Date:		Weight:			

Caliper Measurements

Chest:		Suprillac:		Bicep:	
Subscap:		Thigh:		Calf:	
Abd:		Low Bck:		Tricep:	

Girth Measurements

Shoulders:		Chest:		Waist:		Hips:		L.Bi:	
L Thigh:		R.Thigh:		L.Calf:		R.Calf:		R.Bi:	

Body Fat%:		
Fat Lbs:		
Lean Mass:		

SPARTA FITNESS

NAME: Theresa AGE: 54 TRAINER:

Date:	9/16/15	Height:	5'9"	Weight:	174

Caliper Measurements

Chest:	5	Suprillac:	3	Bicep:	6
Subscap:	11	Thigh:	26	Calf:	14
Abd:	9	Low Bck:	8	Tricep:	12

Girth Measurements

Shoulders:	44	Chest:		Waist:	32	Hips:	40	L.Bi:	
L Thigh:	23 1/2	R.Thigh:	23 1/2	L.Calf:		R.Calf:		R.Bi:	

Body Fat%:	14.59	
Fat Lbs:	25.38	
Lean Mass:	148.62	

Date:	10/9/15	Weight:	167		

Caliper Measurements

Chest:	4	Suprillac:	2	Bicep:	5
Subscap:	9	Thigh:	24	Calf:	14
Abd:	6	Low Bck:	8	Tricep:	11

Girth Measurements

Shoulders:	43 1/2	Chest:		Waist:	30 1/2	Hips:	39 3/4	L.Bi:	
L Thigh:	22 3/4	R.Thigh:	22 3/4	L.Calf:		R.Calf:		R.Bi:	

Body Fat%:	13.42	
Fat Lbs:	22.41	
Lean Mass:	144.59	

Date:	11/9/15	Weight:	162		

Caliper Measurements

Chest:	3	Suprillac:	1	Bicep:	4
Subscap:	9	Thigh:	19	Calf:	10
Abd:	6	Low Bck:	8	Tricep:	10

Girth Measurements

Shoulders:	42 1/2	Chest:		Waist:	30	Hips:	39 1/2	L.Bi:	
L Thigh:	22 1/4	R.Thigh:	22 1/4	L.Calf:		R.Calf:		R.Bi:	

Body Fat%:	11.67	
Fat Lbs:	18.90	
Lean Mass:	143.10	

Appendix B

Basic Workout 30-day Plan

Here is an example of Theresa's 30-day plan:

Day 1
HIIT cardio 30—45 min fasted in early morning
20-30 min core training:

- Bosu Spiderman planks 1—15 reps per side
- Bicycle crunches 10—15 reps per side
- Bosu side planks 10—15 reps per side
- Suspended mountain climbers 30—45 sec repeat 3-6 sets
- Rest period 30—45 seconds after an entire completed set

Day 2:
Upper-body circuit, 45—60min**:**
(5 min shoulder warm-up)

Circuit 1 (shoulder blast) standing or seated

- Dumbbell (DB) front raise 12—15 reps each arm
- DB side laterals 12—15 reps
- DB presses 12—15 reps
- DB upright rows 12—15 reps

Repeat circuit 3 to 5 times
Rest period 30—45 seconds

Next, move to assisted pull ups 3—4 sets of 10—15 reps

Circuit 2 (back and arms)

- High lateral pull-downs 12—15 reps
- Speed rows using band in squatting position 30—45 seconds
- Tricep push-downs on cable machine 15—20 reps
- Standing bicep DB curls 12—15 reps

Repeat circuit 3—5 times
Rest period 30—45 seconds

Circuit 3

- One arm DB row on flat bench 12—15 reps
- Tricep kickbacks using DB 15—20 reps
- Seated concentration DB curls 15—20 each arm

Repeat 3—5 times
Rest period 30—45 seconds

Circuit 4

- Seated cable rows (machine) 12—15 reps
- Standing tricep pushdowns using tubing 30—45 seconds
- Standing curls using tubing 30—45 seconds

Repeat 3—5 times
Rest period 30—45 seconds

Day 3:
Cardio day (HIIT, 30—45 min)

Day 4:
Lower-body circuit (45—60min)

5 min warm-up
Leg extensions 15—20 reps, 4 sets

Circuit 1

- Smith machine squats 15—20 reps
- Walking lunges 50—75 yards
- Seated or kneeling leg curls machine, 15—20 reps

Repeat 3 or 4 sets
Rest period 30—45 seconds

Circuit 2

- Seated leg press (machine) 15—20 reps
- Standing body weight squats 30—40 reps
- Anterior reach lunge, 12—15 each leg

Repeat 4 or 5 times
Rest period 30—45 seconds

Circuit 3

- Jump squats, 30 seconds
- Alternating jumping lunges, 30 seconds

Repeat 3 or 4 times
Rest period 30—45 seconds

Circuit 4

- Lying glute bridge off stability ball, legs straight 15—20 reps
- Lying glute bridge with knees bent, feet flat on ball, pushing hips up as high as you can, 15—20 reps
- Lying leg curls on stability ball, 15—20 reps

Repeat 3 or 4 times
Rest period 30—45 seconds

Day 5	Cardio and core
Day 6	Upper-body circuit
Day 7	Cardio and core
Day 8	Lower-body circuit
Day 9	Cardio and core
Day 10	Upper-body circuit
Day 11	Lower-body circuit
Day 12	Cardio and core
Day 13	Upper-body circuit
Day 14	Cardio and core
Day 15	Lower-body circuit
Day 16	Cardio and core
Day 17	Upper-body circuit
Day 18	Cardio core
Day 19	Cardio core
Day 20	Upper-body circuit
Day 21	Cardio core
Day 22	Lower-body circuit
Day 23	Cardio core
Day 24	Upper-body circuit
Day 25	Lower-body circuit
Day 26	Cardio core
Day 27	Cardio core
Day 28	Upper-body circuit
Day 29	Cardio core
Day 30	Lower-body circuit

Basic Meal Plan

Meal 1 Before workout

1 scoop Iso whey protein shake
1/3 cup oats or cream of rice mixed in shake
1tbsp almond butter/natural peanut butter (blend all together)
You can add berries to sweeten the taste

Meal 2 After workout

2 whole eggs 1 egg white (cage free), 1 oz. baby spinach, 1tsp coconut oil make omelet
⅛ sea salt
¼ avocado

Meal 3

4 oz. grilled chicken or tuna or lean turkey
3 oz. spring mix or baby spinach
½–1 avocado or 1oz walnuts
2 tbsp. balsamic dressing or oil and vinegar
⅛ tsp sea salt

Meal 4

1 scoop Iso whey protein
1 small apple or rice cake
1 tbsp. natural peanut butter or almond butter

Meal 5

4 oz. salmon (1or 2 days a week) chicken breast or lean turkey
6 oz. asparagus or any green vegetable
1 tbsp apple cider vinegar
1 tbsp Udos oil (Made by FLORA and available at HEB by supplements in refrigerator)
⅛ tsp. sea salt or 1 tbsp. salt

Meal 6 (Optional meal, can replace another as well)

3 egg whites, 2 oz. spinach, low fat Parmesan cheese
1 tbsp. coconut oil to cook omelet

Additional Snacks

Homemade guacamole (eat with black bean chips)

1 ripe avocado
Chopped-up garlic clove
Sea salt
1 tsp. chili
1 tbsp. fresh lemon juice

Mash avocado with fork

Homemade salsa (eat with black bean chips)

2 tomatoes, chopped
3 cloves garlic, chopped
Juice of 1 lemon
1 onion, chopped
1 jalapeño pepper, chopped

Mix all ingredients in a large bowl, cover and let sit in the refrigerator a few hours. The longer it sits, the hotter it becomes. Stir before serving.

Homemade hummus

1 medium garlic clove
½ cup sesame tahini
3 tbsp. water
Juice of 2 lemons
16 oz. can of chickpeas, drained and mashed
Sea salt

You can use a mini food processor that holds about four cups to make this. Put the garlic clove in the food processor and chop it. Add the well-mixed tahini sauce (you will probably have to mix this together in the measuring cup because it tends to separate into the nut paste and oil). Add the water and mix it in the processor. It will become a paste. Add the lemon juice until the mixture becomes creamy. Water thickens the mixture, lemon juice thins it.

Wash and drain the chickpeas. Add them a handful at a time to the mixture in the processor, until the whole can has been added. Add salt. Serve on celery sticks.

Recommended Reading

Ageless: The Naked Truth about Bioidentical Hormones **by Suzanne Somers**

A national bestseller and a classic, this real-life guide to bioidentical hormones by the beloved celebrity explains how taking these supplements can change your life. Somers uses her decades of health and wellness experience to explain how hormones impact a woman's health, especially in middle age and after menopause and/or after a hysterectomy, and she shares stories of many women who have been helped by this new category of hormones. She makes it very clear that bioidentical hormones are natural, versus traditional medical hormone therapies, which use synthetic hormones that are not familiar to the human body.

Wheat Belly: Lose the Wheat, Lose the Weight, and Find Your Path Back to Health **by William David MD**

A world-famous cardiologist shows how eliminating wheat from your diet can reverse weight gain, fat storage and unsightly bulges and possibly eradicate a host of common American health problems. He contends that scientific tinkering with wheat and agribusiness over the past three decades have produced a product that is a far cry from what our grandparents ate and is the main cause of the national obesity epidemic, as well as many of our national health issues. He offers a guide to eliminating wheat from your diet, as well as case studies of men and women who have changed their lives and waistlines.

Wheat Belly 30-Minute (or Less) Cookbook: 200 Quick and Simple Recipes to Lose the Wheat, Lose the Weight, and Find Your Path Back to Health **by William David MD**

A companion cookbook to the ground-breaking *Wheat Belly* bestseller with a wealth of quick and delicious recipes to help guide you on your dietary change.

***Against All Grain: Delectable Paleo Recipes to Eat Well & Feel Great* by Danielle Walker**

After suffering from an autoimmune disease for years, this self-taught chef experimented in her own kitchen to reform her diet and create amazingly delicious recipes which she has written up in this bestselling paleo diet cookbook. She has written a follow up volume with an additional 100 recipes that are all grain-free, gluten free and dairy free, *Danielle Walker's Against All Grains: Meals Made Simple: Gluten-Free, Dairy-Free and Paleo Recipes*, as well as two holiday cookbooks, *Danielle Walker's Against All Grain: Joyful 25 Christmas and Holiday Gluten-Free, Grain-Free and Paleo Recipes* and *Danielle Walker's Against All Grain: Thankful, 20 Gluten-Free and Paleo Recipes.*

***The Grain Brain: The Surprising Truth about Wheat, Carbs, and Sugar—Your Brain's Silent Killers* by Dr. David Perlmutter and Kristin Loberg**

This ground-breaking Number 1 *New York Times* bestseller by a neurologist exposes the harmful health consequences of the American diet and wheat, carbs and sugar on the brain. He shares long-suppressed medical evidence about these foods as well as a plan to revitalize the body and the brain. The book was a finalist for a 2013 Books for a Better Life Award.

***The Grain Brain Cookbook: More Than 150 Life-Changing Gluten-Free Recipes to Transform Your Health* by Dr. David Perlmutter**

A companion book to the previous title for those who are serious about changing what and how they eat.

***Fed Up: Understanding How Food Affects Your Child and What You Can Do About It* by Sue Dengate**

A classic first published in 2003, and completely updated and revised in 2011. Dengate found the connection between synthetic food additives and natural chemicals in food and behavior as it relates to children when her own children were suffering from diagnosed ADHD. Her book chronicles how learning difficulties, behavioral problems and minor chronic illness in children and adults might be the result of intolerance to food chemicals. She shares her own elimination diet, as well as personal stories, and those of her friends and colleagues in changing their diets and their lives.

***What it takes to be # 1* by Vince Lomdardi and Vince Lombardi, Jr.**

A classic book for leadership and inspiration from the 1970s, this book never fails to give hope and motivation to anyone who picks it up. Vince Lombardi was the head coach of the Green Bay Packers in the 60s, and his son has added his personal insight to the story of his father's great accomplishments. It has been read by millions over the past 50 years.

***The New Encyclopedia of Modern Body Building, The Bible of Body Building, Fully Updated and Revised* by Arnold Schwarzenegger and Bill Dobbins (2012 edition)**

Arnold inspired an entire generation of bodybuilders and I learned much of my diet and exercise basics and my sense of motivation from this man. His books are still relevant and inspirational, and worth having on your shelf.

Acknowledgements

First, I would like to thank my Heavenly Father for his guidance and patience. He has given me the strength and faith to get through the adversities I have had to overcome in my life. I would also like to thank my son, Michael; my brother, Brian; and my father, Louis, who are looking down on me from heaven, for giving me the courage to pursue my dreams and make them come true.

I would definitely like to thank my wonderful, loving and supportive husband, Lamar, for his constant devotion and strength in letting me be whatever I want to be in this life and never telling me, "No, you can't do that." You have always been a positive partner in our marriage and allowed me to chase my dreams. With you by my side, I can achieve anything!

Thanks to my beautiful daughter, Tashina, and my two beautiful twin grandsons, Zach and Zane, for being the shining lights in my life. You three are the reason I am still on this earth after Michael died, giving me the strength to go on and make a difference in this world to create a legacy for all of us that will be remembered. Without you, I would be an empty shell, so I thank you!

I would also like to thank my family, siblings, my extended family and friends for their continued support and for believing in me through all I have been through and never letting me lose sight of the bigger picture.

There are more of you than I can possibly acknowledge, but you know who you are. This book's very existence is a culmination of friendships and support of many individuals who have impacted my life in one way or another, and I am profoundly grateful to each and every one of you!

I also want to thank my friend, manager and PR rep Paula for allowing me to be who I am, shine like a bright star and not try to change me. It has been refreshing to work with you and have you allow me to be the fluttering butterfly always wanting to chase after more dreams and somehow leave my mark in this world while I am here. You have allowed me to grow and blossom when others wanted to change me. You have seen my vision from day one and have encouraged me to strive for it all. Without you and the amazing Astonish Media team, I would not have been able to be where I am at in such a short period of time. Your friendship has also helped me weather some tough times but also celebrate my achievements. Thank you

These special people, Dr. George Davis, Sean Smith and Heather Smith, were key elements in adding their expertise to this book. I believe like-people attract like-people. Dr. George, I love that I have found a doctor who believes that good health starts with a healthy lifestyle. You have always shared this fabulous belief with me, and together we walk that walk. Sean and Heather Smith are a valuable team that has been truly instrumental in keeping me on course while battling my crazy-busy schedule. Having you both help me strive for physical levels that most people in their 50s would never attempt, because you also believe in that healthy way of life, just makes working with you both a true joy. Having you both as part of my team of life, the healthy eating, the never-ending workouts and understanding the hormonal imbalances women of all ages have to deal with, makes life so much more enjoyable with your incredible knowledge. Without you three people, this book and my life would not be complete!

Last, but not least, I am especially grateful to my publisher Lori Perkins for your ability to choose me as the fitness guru to write this book for you. For your trust and intuition that I was the right person to help make this book a reality and allow me to be free-spirited and never telling me that my ideas were not right. With that, I am grateful that you also allowed my true self to shine through and be totally naked and vulnerable to show women it is okay to be "naked."

About the Author

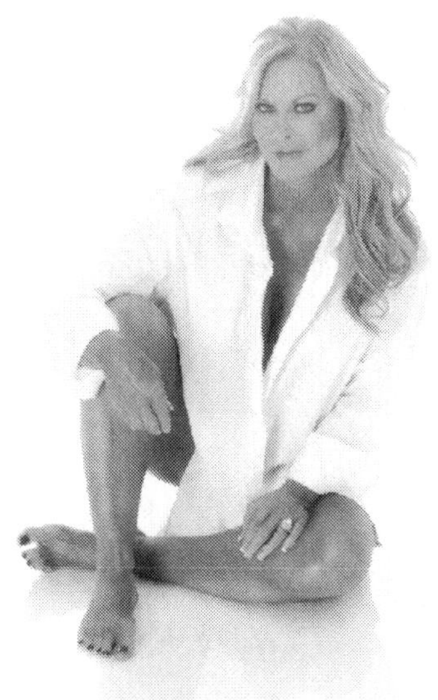

Theresa Roemer is an author, media personality, entrepreneur and small-business owner based in Houston, Texas.

Theresa's passion for health started at a young age. As a child Theresa was diagnosed with rheumatic fever many times over, which caused her to have a heart murmur; she was sickly, and her doctors diagnosed her with a lifetime of physical constraints. Determined to prove the doctors wrong, Theresa began her lifelong journey to stay active, healthy and physically fit. Theresa took the U.S. Open title in bodybuilding at the age of 40 and held the titles of Mrs. Houston U.A., Mrs. Texas U.A., and was the 1st runner up for Mrs. United America concurrently.

Theresa's passion for health inspired her to write *Naked in 30 Days* to empower women to feel as vibrant and healthy at 45 and beyond as they did at 25.

Visit Theresa on:
www.theresaroemer.com, Instagram (Theresa_Roemer),
Facebook (Theresa Roemer), Twitter (@TheresaRoemer)
and YouTube (youtube.com/user/theresaroemer)

Other Riverdale Avenue Books You Might Enjoy

A Star Shattered:
The Rise and Fall and Rise of a Wrestling Diva
By Tamara "Sunny" Sytch

We Love Jenni:
An Unauthorized Biography of Jenni Rivera
By Marc Shapiro

Welcome to Shondaland:
An Unauthorized Biography of Shonda Rhimes
By Marc Shapiro

The Secret Life of E.L. James
By Marc Shapiro

Lorde: Your Heroine
How This Young Feminist Broke the Rules and Succeeded
By Marc Shapiro

Hot Flashes: Adventures in Dating Through Menopause
By Michelle Churchill

Confessions of a Librarian
By Barbara Foster

Made in the USA
San Bernardino, CA
20 March 2016